ATLAS OF
Endometrial
Histopathology

Gisela Dallenbach-Hellweg·Hemming Poulsen

ATLAS OF
Endometrial
Histopathology

Munksgaard / *North and South America:*
Copenhagen / **W. B. SAUNDERS COMPANY**
/ *Philadelphia/London/Toronto*

Atlas of Endometrial Histopathology
1st edition 1st printing 1985
Copyright © 1985 Munksgaard, Copenhagen
All rights reserved

Cover by Lars Thorsen
Composition by Satsform, Åbyhøj
Reproductions by Illugrafia, Herlev
Printed in Denmark 1985 by Jydsk Centraltrykkeri, Århus

ISBN 87-16-09626-6

Distributed in North and South America by W.B. Saunders Company, Philadelphia, Pennsylvania

ISBN 0-7216-1647-x

Library of Congress catalog card No. 8A-52253

Contents

Introduction

The cyclic changes in function and histology of the endometrium and the rapidity with which they take place complicate the histopathologic diagnosis. Disease states of varying intensities that superimpose themselves on these fluctuating functional changes often produce complex admixtures of the functional state and the damage wrought by the pathologic processes.

The pathologist's functional and morphologic diagnoses should represent the result of close cooperation with the attending gynecologist. The prime purpose of this atlas is to help the pathologist to find, classify and diagnose differentially the changes he sees under his microscope. We have kept the text brief. It provides a short description of the pathology of the disease, summarizes and differentiates the causes that come into question, and explains the clinical importance of the condition and thereby how to treat it. Accordingly, this book's approach to diseases is the opposite to that of the textbook which systematically presents the histopathology of the endometrium according to etiology. This atlas proceeds from the histologic changes and relates these to the possible causes. It follows, as it were, the line of thought which the pathologist uses, sparing him the search through different chapters of a textbook on etiology of comparable histologic states. In addition, it obviates duplicating pictures of similar structural changes caused by different diseases.

The atlas is restricted to the endometrium. Neighboring parts of the uterus are included only when we considered them important in differential diagnoses. We have refrained from including electron microscopic pictures since they can be dispensed with in routine diagnostic studies.

This book is intended for all pathologists, to aid them in their routine diagnostic work and to explain as clearly as possible just how comprehensive, complex and important the histopathology of the endometrium has become in the last few years. The book is also meant for the clinician, to help guide him through the broad spectrum of possibilities of histopathologic diagnosis of the endometrium, especially in functional disturbances. If this atlas, through its sharp distinction of histopathologic states, helps to foster improved dialogue between pathologists and clinicians so that optimal therapy of the patients can be provided, then the atlas has fulfilled its purpose.

Gisela Dallenbach-Hellweg and *Hemming Poulsen*
Mannheim and Copenhagen, December 1984

Technical remarks

Selection of the proper time for curettage

In order to obtain optimal diagnostic results, the time for curettage must be carefully selected. In *sterility patients*, the differential diagnosis of the various causes of sterility is best made shortly before the onset of menstruation. Only at this late time can the failure in endometrial differentiation be completely surveyed. In *menorrhagia* possibly due to irregular shedding, the best time for curettage is from 5 to 10 days after the onset of menstruation, in order to recognize remnants of non-lysed mucosa. In *metrorrhagia* curettage is best done without delay when much of the endometrium is still available for examination. With *amenorrhea* in a patient in the reproductive age period, a pregnancy must be excluded before curettage is performed.

Preparation of the endometrial specimen

For *fixation*, a 4% neutral solution of formaldehyde is commonly used and is ideal for most of the diagnostic procedures involved in endometrial examination. Routine *staining* of all specimens should include Hematoxylin-Eosin and a connective tissue stain, for instance van Gieson. The latter is particularly important for recognizing endometrial polyps or portions of them, and hyalinized placental villi. An additional PAS reaction may be helpful in detecting small amounts of glycogen or mucopolysaccharides in glandular epithelial cells. A reticulin impregnation can be useful for verifying tissue lysis or for distinguishing between various types of tumors. These four staining methods suffice for most questions arising in routine examination of the endometrial biopsy.

Interpretation of endometrial specimens

Since the endometrial biopsy may contain admixtures of small pieces from various endometrial layers, its interpretation is more difficult than that of intact endometrium received with a surgically removed uterus. Only the functional layer is of diagnostic value in the recognition of functional disturbances. On the other hand, early adenomatous or carcinomatous changes may best be detected in the basal layer. The isthmus mucosa is unsuited for functional diagnosis; it may give a false impression of atrophy or functional deficiency. Regions of necrosis in curettings may have various causes: they should always be reported. Myomatous proliferations may indicate the presence of submucous leiomyomas as the cause of functional bleeding. If the endometrial biopsy contains only endocervical mucosa, the gynecologist may not have reached the endometrial cavity for various reasons, e.g. stenosis of the isthmus or endocervical canal. If fragments of tissue not occurring in the uterine cavity are found in the endometrial biopsy, e.g. fatty tissue, this finding should raise strong suspicions, if not being indicative, of a perforation of the uterine wall and should therefore always be reported. For further details, see Dallenbach-Hellweg, 1981.

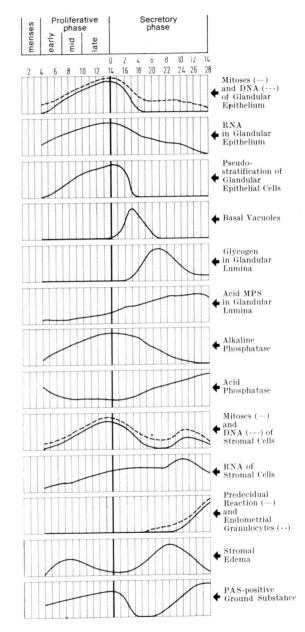

Table 1:
Morphologic criteria important in dating the
endometrial cycle.
(from Dallenbach-Hellweg,G. 1981).

CHAPTER 1

The normal endometrium

The normal menstrual cycle

The proliferative phase

This phase usually lasts fourteen days, but under physiologic conditions may fluctuate between ten and twenty days. It is therefore impossible to distinguish each day during this phase. Consequently, it is subdivided only into the early, middle and late proliferative phases. For clinical purposes this subdivision suffices, since the relevant functional changes become evident only in the secretory phase.

Early proliferative phase (Figs. 1 and 2): The endometrium is low with sparse, narrow and straight glands evenly distributed in a loose stroma of spindle-shaped cells. The glandular epithelial cells are low columnar; they contain small, rounded or oval-shaped chromatindense nuclei in a sparse cytoplasm. The stromal cells are poorly differentiated, of equal size with small, dense nuclei in a scanty cytoplasm. Nucleoli are inconspicuous and mitoses are very rare. The cells are surrounded by a firm reticulin network. Spiral arterioles are undeveloped. The surface epithelium is flat and still regenerating.

Clinical possibilities: a) 4th to 7th day of a normal menstrual cycle. b) Anovulatory cycle with follicular insufficiency. c) Deficient proliferation, when patient is beyond the 7th day of her cycle, or postmenopausal.

Distinction is possible only by precise statement of the day of the menstrual cycle and by recording (in anovulatory cycles) the basal body temperature curve. Distinction on morphologic grounds alone is not possible.

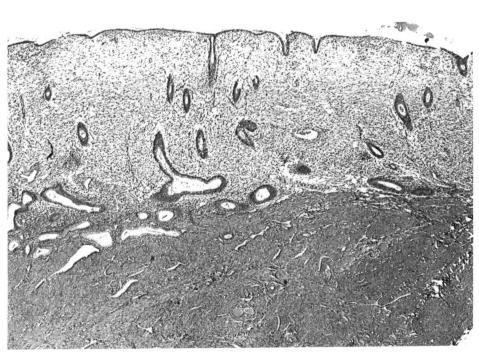

Fig. 1. Early proliferative phase. H & E, ×25.

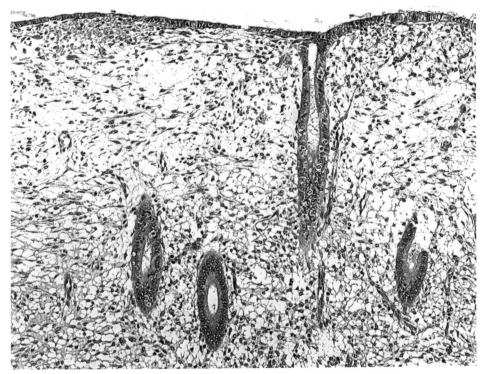

Fig. 2. Early proliferative phase. H & E, ×100.

Mid proliferative phase (Figs. 3 and 4): Here there is beginning tortuosity of glands due to their increase in length, which exceeds the growth in height of the endometrium. The glandular epithelial cells are tall columnar and contain slightly enlarged oval-shaped, chromatin-rich nuclei in a dense, sparse cytoplasm rich in RNA. Nucleoli are prominent, mitoses frequent. The spindle-shaped stromal cells are still poorly differentiated, but rich in DNA and RNA with occasional mitoses and separated by interstitial edema. Spiral arterioles are not seen. The surface epithelium has increased in height and is now low columnar.

Clinical possibilities: a) 8th to 11th day of a normal menstrual cycle. b) Anovulatory cycle.

Distinction is possible only by precise statement of the day of the menstrual cycle and by recording (in anovulatory cycles) the basal body temperature curve.

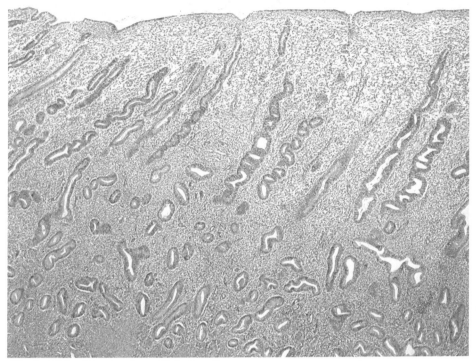

Fig. 3. Midproliferative phase. H & E, ×25.

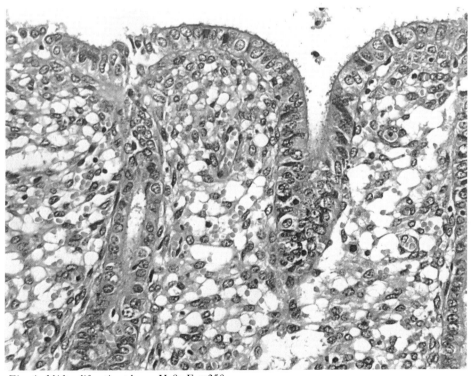

Fig. 4. Midproliferative phase. H & E, ×250.

15

Late proliferative phase (Figs. 5, 6 and 7): There is marked tortuosity of glands, which are lined by tall columnar epithelial cells piled up against one another with their nuclei at different levels, giving a pseudostratified appearance. The nuclei are enlarged still further, rich in DNA and more elongated or oval-shaped. Nucleoli are quite prominent; mitoses are frequent. The cytoplasm is still sparse and poorly differentiated but rich in RNA. The stromal cells are further enlarged and contain increased amounts of DNA and RNA. They are still of uniform size and without signs of differentiation. Stromal mitoses are frequent. The stromal edema has subsided. The reticulin network is dense. Spiral arterioles are still absent. The general height may be slightly lower than that of the midproliferative phase due to decrease of edema. The surface epithelium is distinctly columnar.

Clinical possibilities: a) 12th to 14th day of a normal menstrual cycle. b) Anovulatory cycle with follicular persistence.

Distinction is possible only by precise statement of the day of the menstrual cycle and by recording (in anovulatory cycles) the basal body temperature curve.

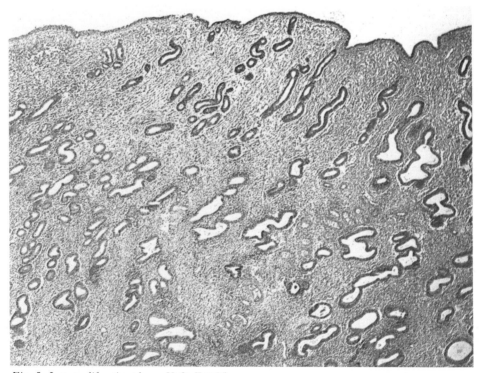

Fig. 5. Late proliferative phase. H & E, ×25.

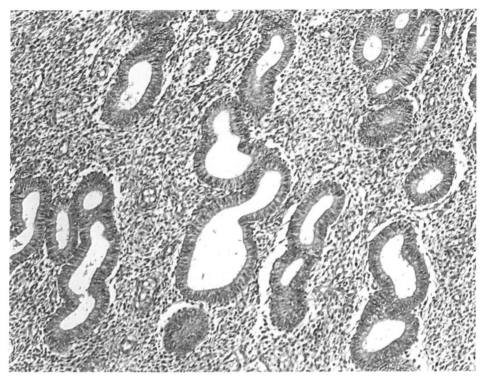

Fig. 6. Late proliferative phase. H & E, ×100.

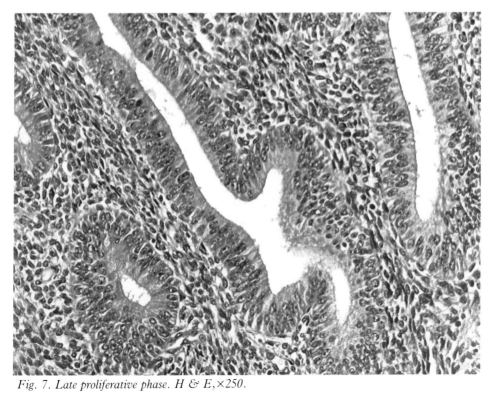

Fig. 7. Late proliferative phase. H & E, ×250.

The secretory phase

In the presence of a normally developing and involuting corpus luteum this phase lasts precisely fourteen days (±one day; Rock and Hertig 1944). If the deviation from this limit is more than two days, a functional disturbance should be diagnosed. The daily changes induced in the endometrium by the influence of progesterone enable us to date the endometrium (Noyes et al. 1950; Moricard 1954; Philippe et al. 1965; Dallenbach and Dallenbach-Hellweg 1968; Table 1). Because the glandular epithelium reacts more quickly to the influence of progesterone than do the stromal cells, a histologic dating is based mainly on the changes of the glandular epithelium during the first week of the secretory phase and on the changes in the stromal cells during the second week. The histologic signs induced in the endometrium by hormones are never uniform. Differences are related to various factors, such as local blood supply, cellular nutrition and various metabolic factors, e.g. receptors for estrogen and progesterone. For dating the endometrium, those regions showing the most advanced changes are relevant. For the clinical interpretation of the individual cycle days see p. 11.

The first day after ovulation is morphologically mute because it takes thirty-six to forty-eight hours before changes induced by the progesterone secretion can be detected with assurance under the light microscope. Sporadic vacuoles appear in some of the glandular cells even right before ovulation but are unreliable as definite signs of ovulation.

The second day after ovulation (Figs. 8 and 9): Numerous basal glycogen vacuoles have now appeared in the glandular epithelium (at least in 50% of the glandular cells). They have pushed the nucleus towards the lumen. By their formation the previously pseudostratified appearance of the nuclei disappears; the nuclei again form a single row. They are still oval-shaped and chromatin-dense. With this new arrangement of the nuclei the glands become increasingly tortuous and enlarge their surfaces at the glandular lumen. Basal vacuoles, however, fail to appear in the superficial portions of the gland where it merges with the surface epithelium (Fig. 9). The surface epithelium of the endometrium remains tall with no signs of basal secretion. No remarkable changes can be detected in the stroma when compared with those of the late proliferative phase.

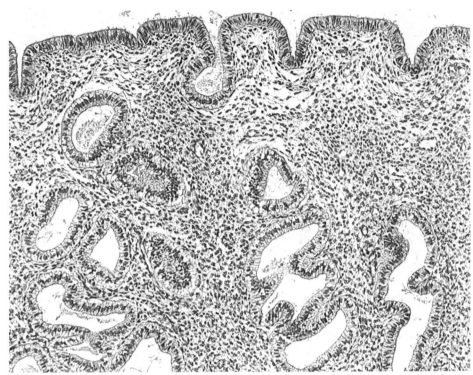

Fig. 8. 2nd day after ovulation. H & E, ×100.

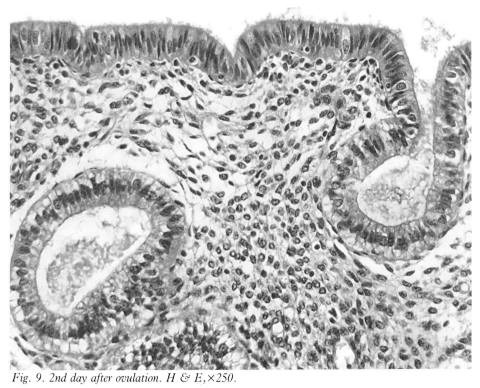

Fig. 9. 2nd day after ovulation. H & E, ×250.

The third day after ovulation (Figs. 10 and 11) shows enlarged basal vacuoles now occupying all glandular epithelial cells. This secretion has pushed all nuclei towards the apical end of the cell where they form a uniform row around the lumen. The nuclei remain dense, rich in chromatin, and only a few mitoses are seen. The cytoplasm still contains abundant RNA.

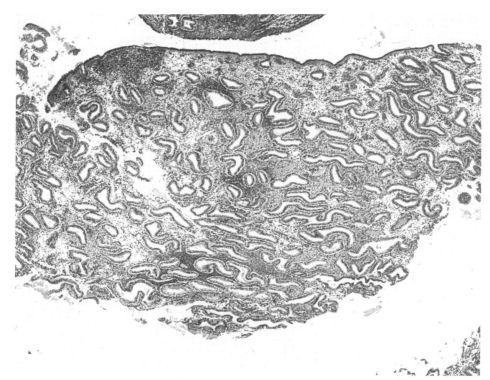

Fig. 10. 3rd day after ovulation. H & E,×25.

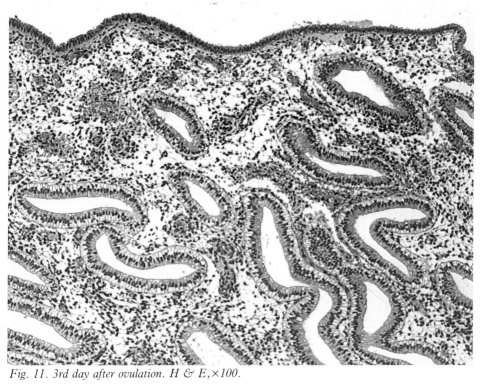

Fig. 11. 3rd day after ovulation. H & E,×100.

21

The fourth day after ovulation (Figs. 12, 13 and 14): The nuclei of the glandular epithelial cells have now become distinctly rounded and less chromatin-dense. A few of them start to return to the base of their cells while tiny amounts of glycogen move towards the lumen. A small rim of mucopolysaccharides can be observed at the luminal margin of the epithelial cells but only with special stains (Fig. 14). This rim is characteristic for the fourth day after ovulation.

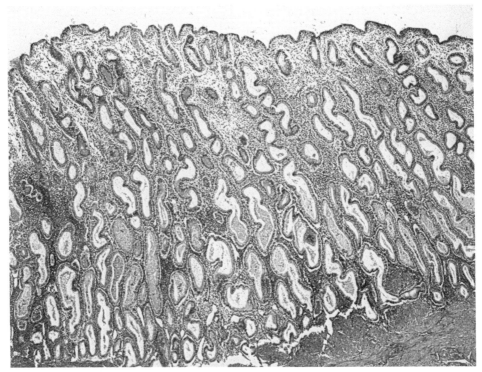

Fig. 12. 4th day after ovulation. H & E, ×25.

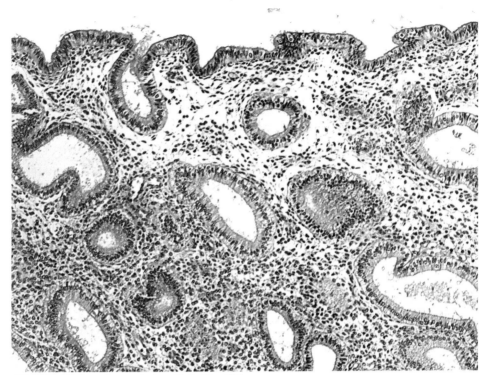

Fig. 13. 4th day after ovulation. H & E, ×100.

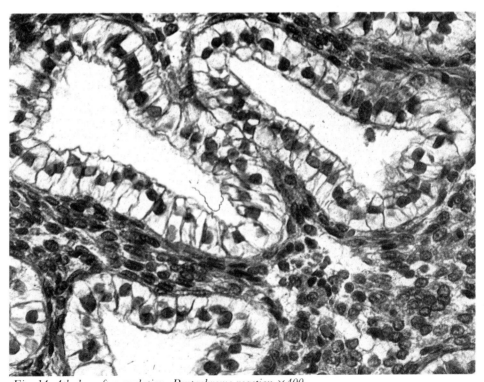

Fig. 14. 4th day after ovulation. Pentachrome reaction, ×400.

The fifth day after ovulation (Fig. 15): The majority of the nuclei in the glandular epithelial cells have now returned to the base of their cells and are distinctly rounded. The glycogen has moved or is moving towards the lumen of the cells on both sides of the nucleus, and beginning secretion can be seen as tiny globular caps at the free margin of the cells. The movement of the glycogen can best be followed with a PAS-stain. Since the nuclei are now vesicular and pale upon staining, they can be easily distinguished from the dense, elongated, basally located nuclei of the cells before the glycogen vacuoles appeared. The nucleoli have become greatly enlarged.

The sixth day after ovulation (Figs. 16 and 17) shows a dilatation of the glandular lumina produced by the continued secretion of glycogen. All epithelial nuclei have now returned to the base of the cells. The glandular cells have decreased in height and their luminal margins appear shredded and hazy due to the excessive apocrine secretion. The RNA content of the cytoplasm is decreased.

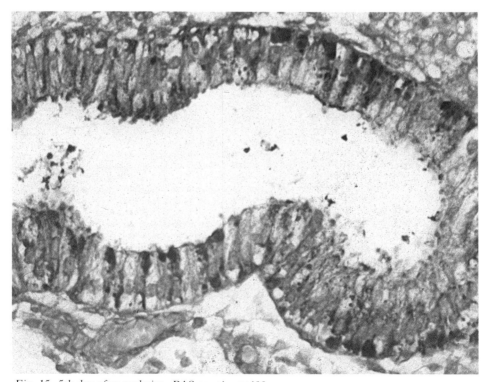

Fig. 15. 5th day after ovulation. PAS-reaction, ×400.

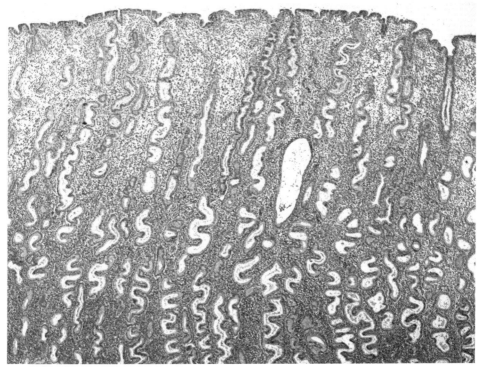

Fig. 16. 6th day after ovulation. H & E, ×25.

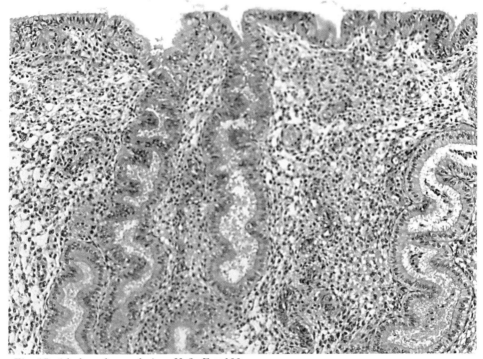

Fig. 17. 6th day after ovulation. H & E, ×100.

The seventh day after ovulation (Figs. 18 and 19): The dilated glandular lumen is now filled with glycogen, which is partly dissolved in H & E stained preparations, giving the lumen a false empty appearance. As a sign of active secretion, the apical ends of the glandular cells appear frayed. No new glycogen is secreted from the cell base. The first stromal reaction after ovulation has occurred and becomes apparent on this day: there is a patchy re-accumulation of stromal edema.

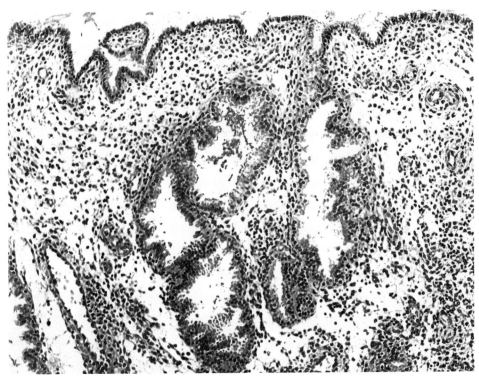

Fig. 18. 7th day after ovulation. H & E, ×100.

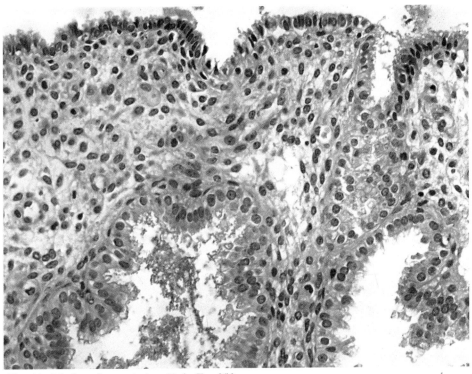

Fig. 19. 7th day after ovulation. H & E, ×250.

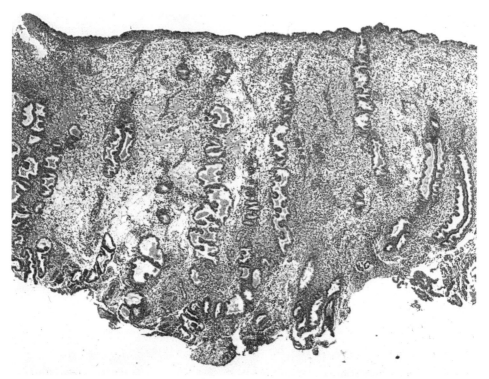

Fig. 20. 8th day after ovulation. H & E, ×25.

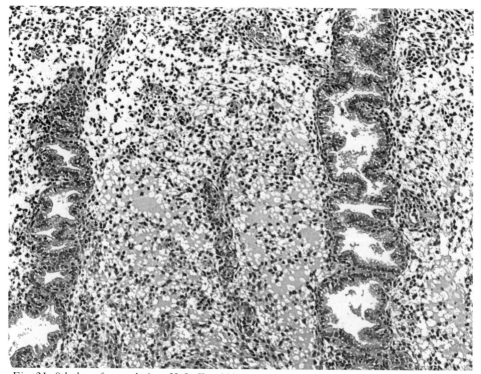

Fig. 21. 8th day after ovulation. H & E, ×100.

The eighth day after ovulation (Figs. 20, 21 and 22): Whereas there is virtually no change in the glandular epithelium compared with the preceding day, stromal edema has reached its maximum for the secretory phase. It is now diffuse and quite intense with the stromal cells widely separated from one another. These are still spindle-shaped but somewhat enlarged. Their differentiation becomes apparent from this day on (Fig. 22). The overall height of the endometrium has increased.

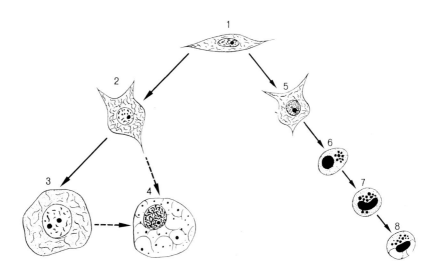

Fig. 22. Schematic drawing of endometrial stromal differentiation (from Dallenbach-Hellweg 1981). 1. Poorly differentiated stromal cell. 2. Stromal cell becoming larger and more globular. 3. Decidual cell. 4. Foamy decidual cell laden with metachromatic granules. 5. Stromal cell becoming smaller and more rounded. 6,7,8. Various stages in the development of endometrial granulocytes.

The ninth day after ovulation (Figs. 23, 24 and 25): The stromal edema has slightly subsided but is still distinct. Groups of spiral arterioles are now prominent. The stromal cells surrounding these spiral arterioles grow larger and more rounded. Their nuclei enlarge and appear less chromatin-dense. Their cytoplasm is increased in amount and in RNA content. The stromal cells which are further away from the arterioles remain only slightly enlarged. Glandular secretion has ceased, but remnants of secreted substance may be found in the glandular lumina.

The tenth day after ovulation (Figs. 26, 27, 28 and 29): At this time two distinct layers of the endometrium can be distinguished under low magnification: The upper compact layer, consisting mainly of stromal cells, and the lower spongious layer, containing distended tortuous glands with serrated edges, exhausted glandular epithelial cells and remnants of inspissated secretion in the wide glandular lumina. The stromal cells around the spiral arterioles have developed into either predecidual cells with large, round, clear nuclei and abundant cytoplasm, or stromal granulocytes with dense, indented or kidney-shaped nuclei and phloxinophilic granules in their cytoplasm (Hamperl 1954; Hellweg 1954) (Fig. 29) which in addition is rich in RNA. These two types of differentiated stromal cells are present in almost equal numbers. This differentiation has only taken place adjacent to the arterial blood supply whereas regions further away have as yet not participated. At this time a sheet-like predecidual change develops in the compact layer of the endometrium.

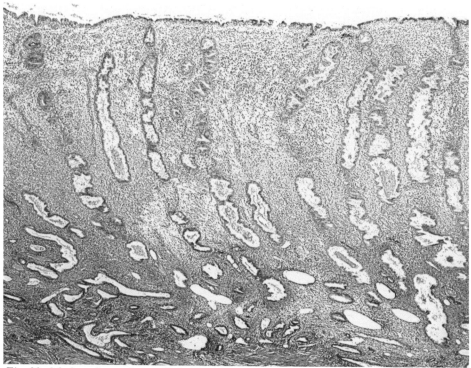

Fig. 23. 9th day after ovulation. H & E, ×25.

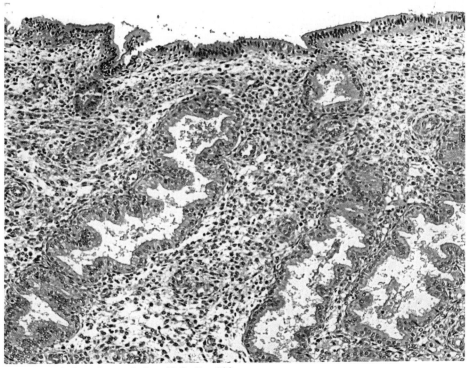

Fig. 24. 9th day after ovulation. H & E, ×100.

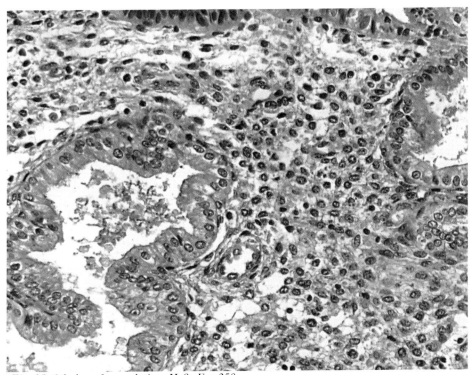

Fig. 25. 9th day after ovulation. H & E, ×250.

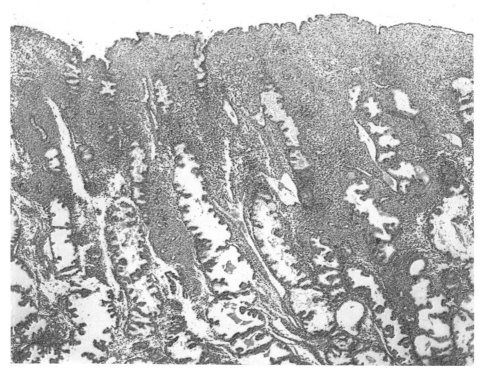

Fig. 26. 10th day after ovulation. H & E,×25.

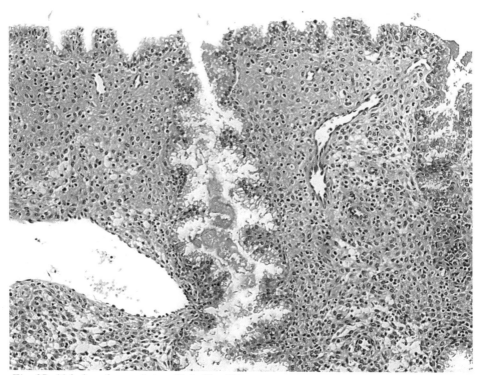

Fig. 27. 10th day after ovulation. H & E,×100.

32

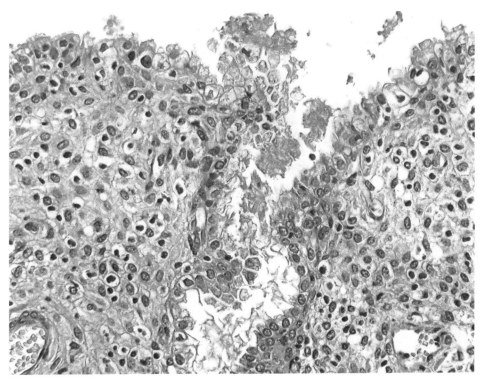

Fig. 28. 10th day after ovulation. H & E, ×250.

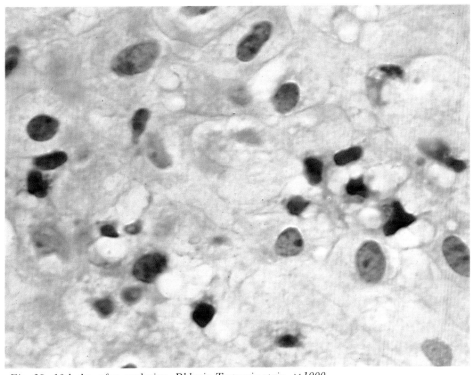

Fig. 29. 10th day after ovulation. Phloxin-Tartrazin stain, ×1000.

The eleventh day after ovulation (Figs. 30, 31 and 32) shows a complete predecidual and granulocytic change of the stromal cells in the compact layer with no remaining undifferenti- ated stromal cells. The surface epithelium has gradually become lower over the previous few days and now appears cuboidal with slightly rounded nuclei.

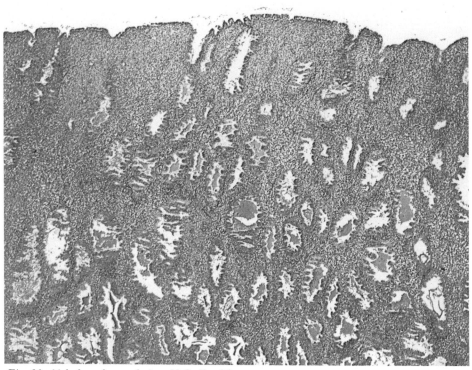

Fig. 30. 11th day after ovulation. H & E, ×25.

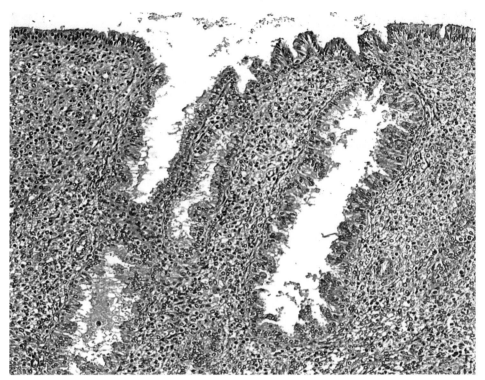

Fig. 31. 11th day after ovulation. H & E,×100.

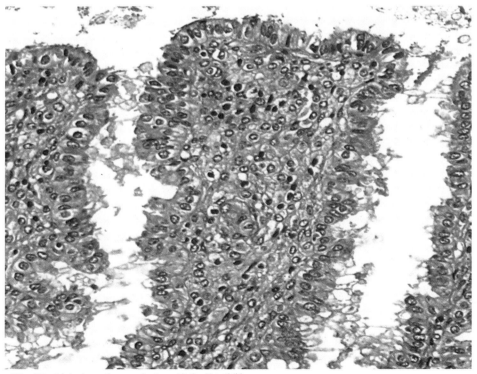

Fig. 32. 11th day after ovulation. H & E,×250.

The twelfth day after ovulation (Figs. 33 and 34): There is the beginning of a decrease in the general height of the endometrium with shrinkage and collapse of the glands, while the stroma loses its edema, becomes dense and remains well differentiated.

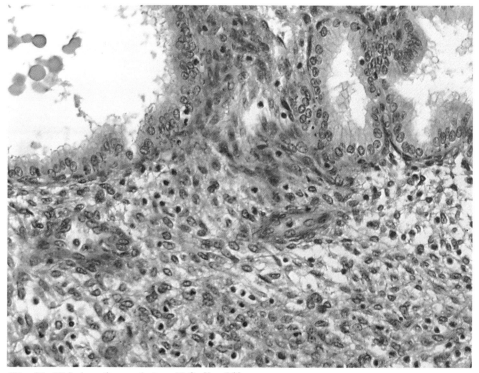

Fig. 33. 12th day after ovulation. H & E, ×250.

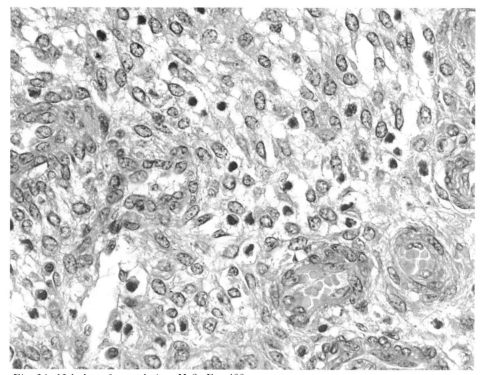

Fig. 34. 12th day after ovulation. H & E, ×400.

The thirteenth day after ovulation (Figs. 35 and 36) shows extensive shrinkage in the overall height of the endometrium. The collapsed glands present a saw-toothed appearance. The predecidual stroma is now very dense. The RNA content in the glandular epithelial cells has diminished, whereas the stromal cells still contain large amounts of RNA.

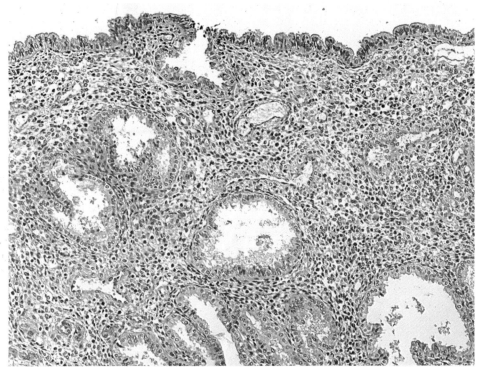

Fig. 35. 13th day after ovulation. H & E, ×100.

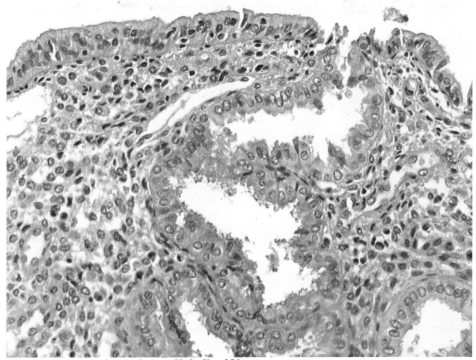

Fig. 36. 13th day after ovulation. H & E, ×250.

The fourteenth day after ovulation (Figs. 37, 38 and 39) shows a very marked delineation between the upper compact layer and the lower spongious layer of the endometrium (Fig. 37). The glandular lumina in the compact layer are narrow, the lining epithelium is low cuboidal and appears inactive, whereas the lumina of the glands in the spongious layer are still saw-toothed and lined by exhausted epithelial cells with a clear cytoplasm now almost devoid of RNA. The glandular cell nuclei reveal a marked decrease in their DNA content. A beginning dissociation of the stromal cells becomes apparent in the compact layer, particularly close to the surface epithelium and around the spiral arterioles, due to the beginning of a dissolution of reticulin fibers. This is caused by secretion of relaxin from the endometrial granulocytes that sets in immediately before menstruation (Dallenbach and Dallenbach-Hellweg 1964). The endometrial granulocytes, which have lost their granules, can be recognized only by their characteristic lobulated nuclei and their vacuolated cytoplasm. The surface epithelium is low and appears inactive.

Clinical possibilities for the entire secretory phase: a) Normal secretory phase, if it corresponds to the day of the menstrual cycle. b) Deficient secretory phase with coordinated true delay, if the day of the menstrual cycle is 3-10 days further advanced than the histologic differentiation. c) Normal secretory phase in amenorrhea due to silent menstruation (Philippe et al. 1966).

Distinction is possible only by precise statement of the day of the menstrual cycle and/or recording of the basal body temperature curve.

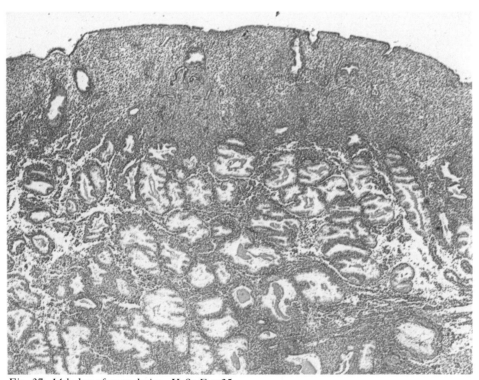

Fig. 37. 14th day after ovulation. H & E, ×25.

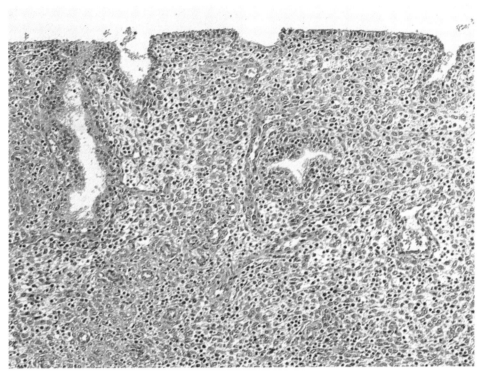

Fig. 38. 14th day after ovulation. H & E, ×100.

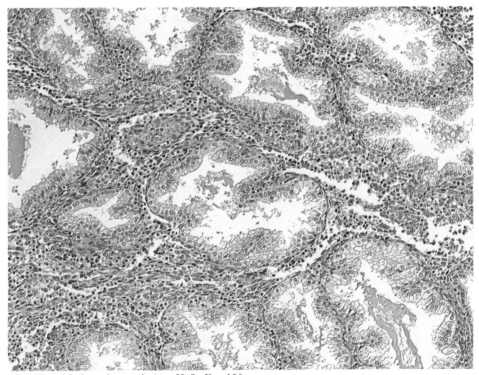

Fig. 39. 14th day after ovulation. H & E, ×100.

Menstruation

The first day of menstruation (Figs. 40, 41 and 42) is characterized by dissociation of glands and stroma and by hemorrhage into the superficial layer corresponding to the compact layer as far as the development of the stromal granulocytes. The dissociated cells still show their predecidual change. The granulocytes have lost their relaxin granules. The surface epithelium is still intact (Fig. 41). The collapsed glands contain remnants of previous secretion. From their structure it is possible, even after the onset of menstruation, to diagnose that ovulation has taken place. The lower portion of the endometrium shows no disintegration of stroma and glands but only shrinkage (Fig. 42). The remaining intact portions participate in the restoration of the endometrium during the next cycle (Sengel and Stoebner 1970).

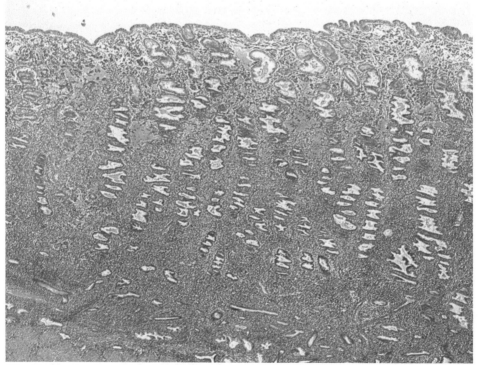

Fig. 40. Menstruation, 1st day. H & E, ×25.

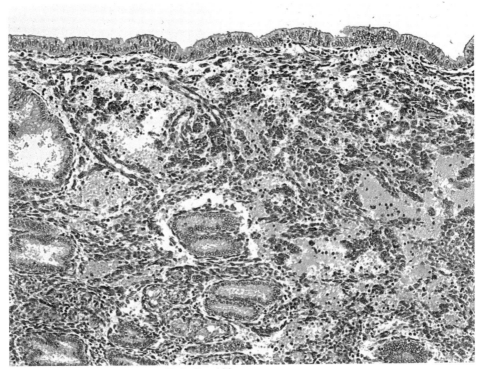

Fig. 41. Menstruation, 1st day. H & E, ×100.

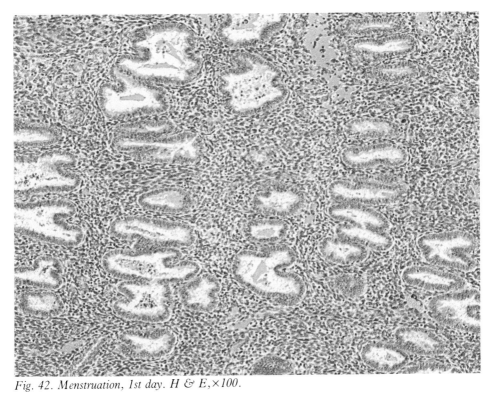

Fig. 42. Menstruation, 1st day. H & E, ×100.

The second day of menstruation (Figs. 43, 44 and 45) shows extensive disintegration and demarcation of those portions of the endometrium which are shed, while the more basal portions remain intact. Scattered degenerating stromal cells and remnants of glandular epithelium lie admixed in unclotted blood and aggregates of polymorphonuclear cells (Flowers and Wilborn 1978).

Clinical correlation of both days: Normal menstruation.

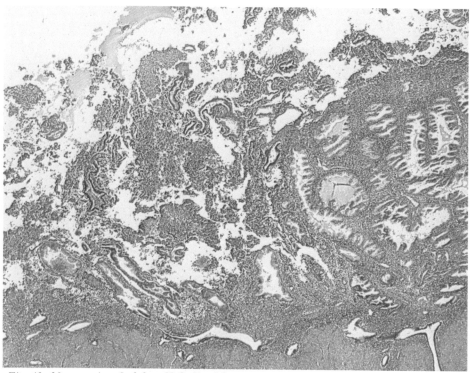

Fig. 43. Menstruation, 2nd day. H & E, ×25.

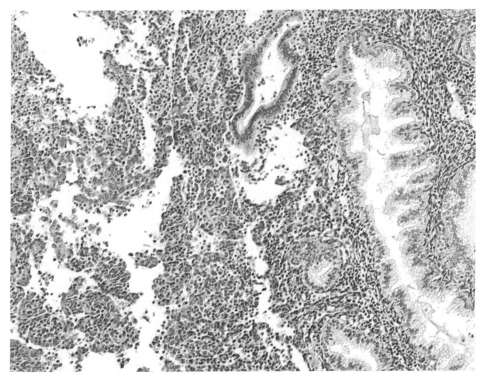

Fig. 44. Menstruation, 2nd day. H & E, ×100.

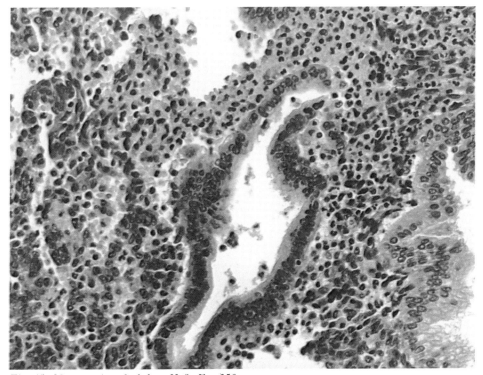

Fig. 45. Menstruation, 2nd day. H & E, ×250.

45

Regeneration

(Figs. 46 and 47). The endometrium is very low and consists mainly of the basal remnants of glands and stroma which are partly re-epithelialized while neighboring areas are still denuded (Nogales et el. 1969, 1978). Stromal cells do not take part in the regeneration. In the epithelial cells the nuclear DNA and cytoplasmic RNA are again increasing, but mitoses are still absent (Ferenczy 1976).

Clinical possibilities: Regeneration after normal menstruation, anovulatory cycle, ovulatory functional disturbances, or after curettage.

Distinction is (except for the regeneration after curettage) not possible at this early stage. When a functional diagnosis is desired by the clinician, the curettage should be repeated later in the cycle, preferably during the late secretory phase.

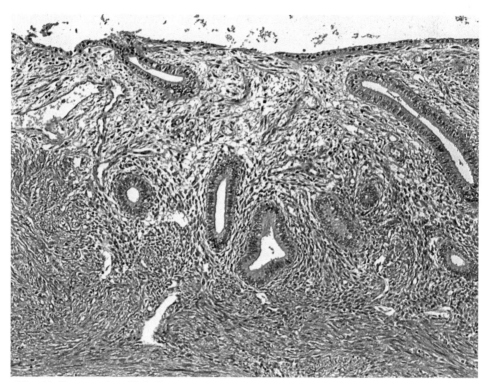

Fig. 46. Regeneration. H & E,×100.

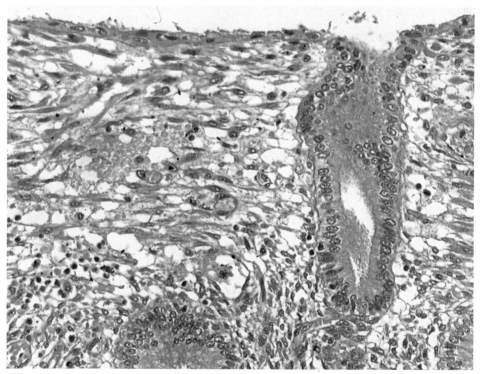

Fig. 47. Regeneration. H & E,×250.

Physiologic variations in the climacterium

The proliferative phase (Fig. 48) shows variations in the width of some glands, although most of the glands are still normal in size, shape and arrangement. The height of the glandular epithelium may vary somewhat.

The secretory phase (Fig. 49) shows slight underdevelopment of some of the glands; these are poorly convoluted and lined by a low cuboidal, rather inactive epithelium with dense small nuclei, whereas the epithelium of neighboring glands is normally differentiated according to the day of the cycle. The general height of the endometrium varies slightly from one region to another. In the lower layers the stroma may be poorly differentiated.

Clinical possibilities: a) Proliferative or secretory phase with climacteric variations. b) Very early stage of irregular proliferation or deficient or irregular secretion when the patient is below age 40.

Distinction is possible by the age of the patient and the menstrual history.

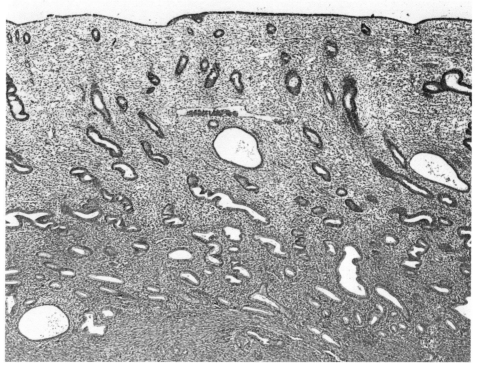

Fig. 48. Physiologic variation of the proliferative phase in the climacterium. H & E,×25.

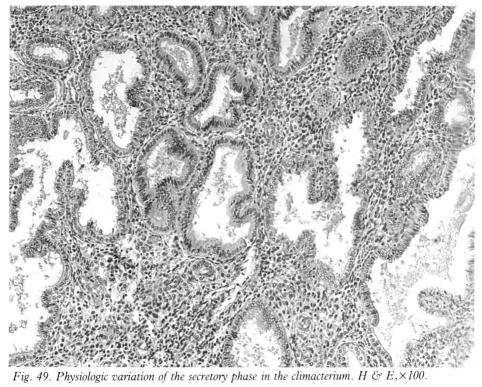

Fig. 49. Physiologic variation of the secretory phase in the climacterium. H & E,×100.

The isthmus mucosa

(Figs. 50 and 51). This portion of the uterine mucosa located between endocervix and endometrium is uniformly flat and consists of slender, often horizontally directed, slit-like glands surrounded by a dense fibrous stroma of small spindle-shaped cells (Fig. 50). The surface and glandular epithelium is low cuboidal and inactive. It does not participate in cyclic changes of either the endocervical or the endometrial type. Occasionally in the isthmus some glands of the endocervical type can be found lined by tall columnar, mucus-secreting epithelium among inactive glands of the endometrial type. The endocervical type of glands may be cystically dilated occasionally (Fig. 50).

Morphologic differential diagnosis: Basal endometrium: The glands of the basal layer branch more, show various degrees of proliferative changes, and their supporting stroma is more irregular since the collagen fibers anchoring the basalis to the myometrium extend in all directions.

Endometrial atrophy: The glands of the atrophic endometrium are much smaller and their lining epithelium is flat. They are surrounded by a dense stroma of small cells devoid of distinctive fibers.

Deficient proliferation: Whereas the glands of the isthmus mucosa may be similar to those of deficient proliferation, the general height of the isthmus mucosa is much lower, and the tangential arrangement of the isthmus glands differs from the perpendicular course of the proliferating glands in deficient proliferation.

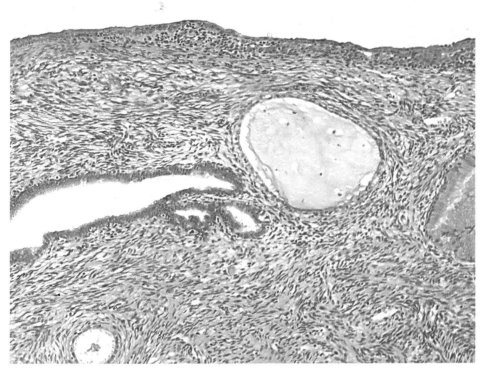

Fig. 50. Isthmus mucoca, H & E, ×100.

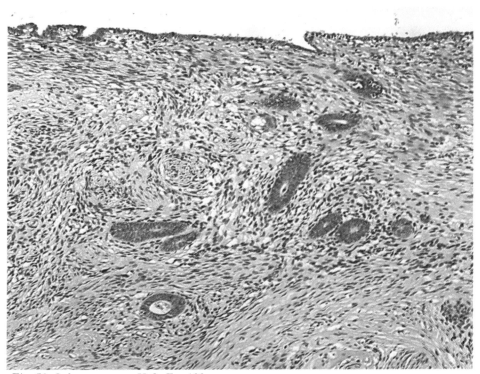

Fig. 51. Isthmus mucosa, H & E, ×100.

CHAPTER 2

Metaplastic changes

The endometrial epithelium may be replaced focally, seldom diffusely, by any other epithelium of Müllerian type. The same holds true for the endometrial stromal cells.

Epithelial metaplasia

Squamous metaplasia and ichthyosis

Squamous metaplasia (Figs. 52-55): Nodules of squamous epithelium arise from the glandular epithelium of irregularly proliferating or cystically dilated hyperplastic glands. Such nodules may develop focally or diffusely and may be found in all endometrial layers (cf. Fig. 103). All transitional stages are encountered, between a few small nodules to extensive metaplasia, which may also involve the surface epithelium, ichthyosis. When the surface epithelium becomes involved (Fig. 52) there is no sharp line of distinction between extensive squamous metaplasia and ichthyosis.

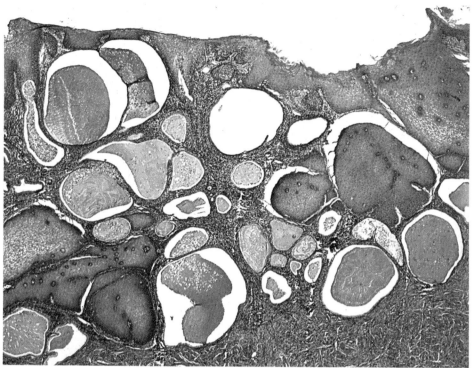

Fig. 52. Squamous metaplasia and ichthyosis. H & E, ×25.

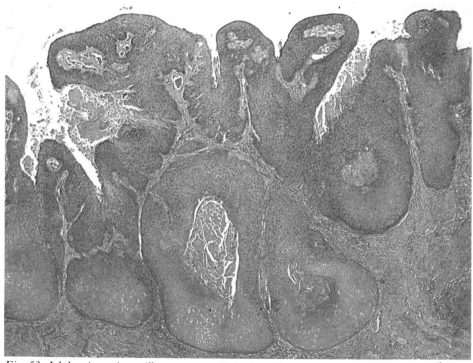

Fig. 53. Ichthyosis uteri, papillary structure. H & E, ×25.

Ichthyosis: In senile atrophy the surface epithelium may alone undergo metaplasia, which is then called ichthyosis. Such a sheet-like surface metaplasia may be smooth or papillary (Fig. 53), normally stratified and mature, occasionally covered with keratinized cells (Fig. 54), or may show loss of stratification with cellular irregularity, depolarization and enlargement of nuclei with occasional mitoses, thus representing epithelial dysplasia (Fig. 55). The underlying endometrium is usually very low, consisting only of small spindle-shaped stromal cells without glands, or containing a very few atrophic glandular remnants. The stroma may contain chronic inflammatory infiltrates comprising mainly lymphocytes and plasma cells (Fig. 55).

Morphologic differential diagnosis: Foci or nodules of squamous metaplasia can be found in glandular cystic or adenomatous hyperplasia and in adenoacanthoma. Sheets of squamous epithelium found as components of curettings are always suspect of carcinoma, regardless of their stage of differentiation. Well-differentiated stratified squamous epithelium may occasionally line the uterine cavity and grow over a mucoepidermoid adenocarcinoma in a postmenopausal woman. On the other hand, an ichthyosis over a senile atrophic endometritis may become dysplastic, probably as a reaction to injury or inflammation without underlying malignancy. Therefore, a thorough fractionated curettage is always required to determine the origin of ichthyosis.

Clinical possibilities and differential diagnosis: a) Individual reaction to long-standing endogenous or exogenous unopposed hyperestrogenism. b) Heterotopic metaplasia of Müllerian origin. c) Reactive squamous cell metaplasia following IUD-induced or senile ulcerative endometritis that covers the defect. d) Superficial portion of a well differentiated mucoepidermoid or squamous cell carcinoma.

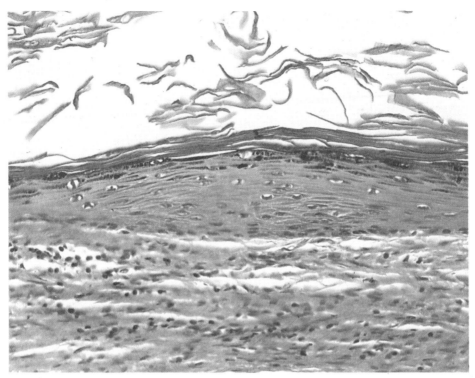

Fig. 54. Ichthyosis uteri, with superficial keratinization. H & E,×250.

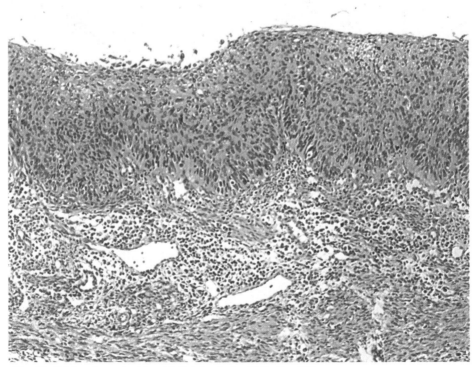

Fig. 55. Ichthyosis uteri with epithelial dysplasia. H & E,×100.

Endocervical metaplasia

(Figs. 56 and 57). Within a proliferating endometrium small neighboring groups or larger areas of glands are found lined by high columnar mucinous epithelium of the mature endocervical type with small dense nuclei at the cellular base. The abundant cytoplasm of the cells is pale in H & E stains and strongly mucin-positive with the PAS reaction. These groups of glands are usually located close to the basal layer and are not shed with menstruation. The surrounding endometrial glands are irregularly proliferated or occasionally cystically dilated, indicative of a distinct estrogenic effect. The stroma is evenly spindle-celled in all regions. The metaplastic glands show an arrangement similar to normal glands, but may occasionally be crowded or convoluted.

Morphologic differential diagnosis: These metaplastic glands must be differentiated from the pale glands in grade 3 (advanced) adenomatous hyperplasia with or without early stromal invasion, where the nuclei are large, depolarized and aneuploid.

Clinical possibilities and differential diagnosis: Endocervical metaplasia a) is usually associated with hyperestrogenism and frequently accompanied by irregular proliferation or glandular cystic hyperplasia. b) Results from heterotopic differentiation of Müllerian epithelium, genetic or reactive.

Distinction is possible by correlation with the functional diagnosis of the endometrium.

Ciliated cell metaplasia

This type of metaplasia resembles the mucosal lining of the Fallopian tube. These foci consist of single-layered or pseudostratified tall columnar ciliated cells with eosinophilic, often vacuolated cytoplasm and may form intraglandular papillae. They occur in proliferative or hyperplastic endometrium during estrogen stimulation. Since occasional ciliated cells are normal constituents of the endometrium, only larger accumulations of these cells should be called metaplasia.

Clinical possibilities and morphologic differential diagnosis: The same as in endocervical metaplasia.

Rare forms of metaplasia of endometrial glandular epithelium

These include clear cells as possible precursors of ciliated cells or eosinophilic (onkocytic) cells. Such cells, however, may not always be truly metaplastic but instead functional variations of glandular cells or cells in disturbed mitosis (see p. 78).

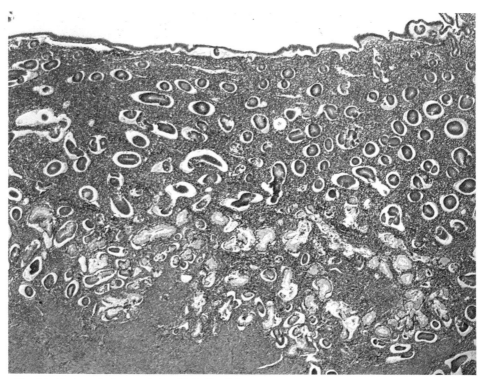

Fig. 56. Endocervical metaplasia, H & E, ×25.

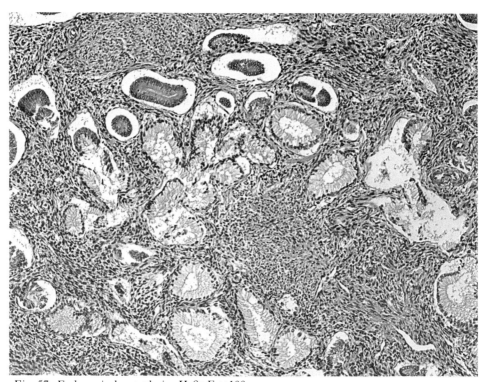

Fig. 57. Endocervical metaplasia. H & E, ×100.

Stromal metaplasia

In rare instances the endometrial stromal cells undergo metaplastic changes. Small foci of smooth muscle metaplasia may occasionally be observed (Fig. 58). Cartilagenous, osseous or fatty metaplasia has rarely been found.

Morphologic differential diagnosis is necessary from: a) Fetal remnants; the metaplastic cells merge with normal stromal cells at their periphery, they do not react as foreign inclusions or growths. b) Mixed mesenchymal tumors by their minimal size and by their benign histologic appearance.

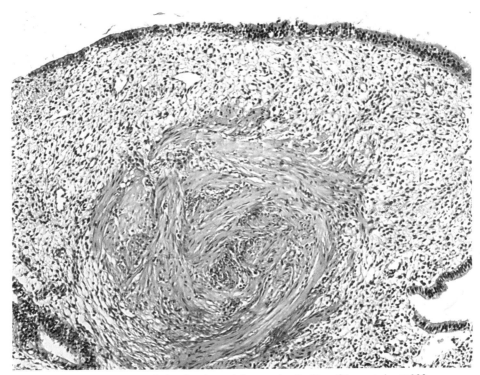

Fig. 58. Smooth muscle metaplasia of endometrial stromal cells, Van Gieson stain, ×100.

CHAPTER 3

Circulatory disturbances

Pathologic edema

(Figs. 59 and 60). The endometrial glands are widely separated and the stromal cells pushed apart by small lakes of edema fluid or diffuse accumulation of edema between them. The reticulin fibers are extremely scanty and also pushed far apart. The small lymphatic channels in the stroma are distended. The appearance of glandular and stromal cells is otherwise within normal limits.

Morphologic differential diagnosis: Pathologic edema must be differentiated from physiologic variations in the vascular and lymphatic circulation during the normal menstrual cycle.

Stromal edema is physiologic in the mid-proliferative phase and on the 22nd day of the normal menstrual cycle (8th day after ovulation).

Clinical possibilities and differential diagnosis: a) Venous or lymphatic obstruction. b) Hormonal dysfunction with endogenous hyperestrogenism. c) Focal variation in hormone supply under exogenic hormones. d) Mechanical pressure on lymphatic vessels by malposition of the uterus, submucous fibromyomas or polyps.

Distinction is possible by correlation of edema with accompanying functional diagnosis of the endometrium and/or surrounding endomyometrium, and with the clinical history.

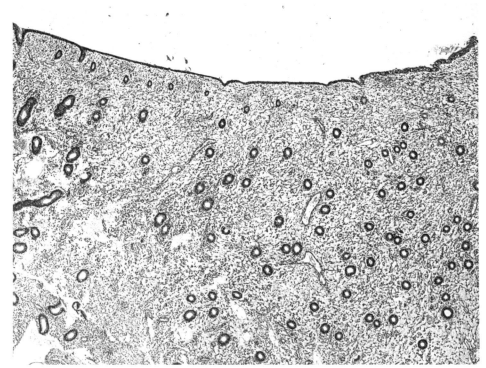

Fig. 59. Pathologic edema. H & E,×25.

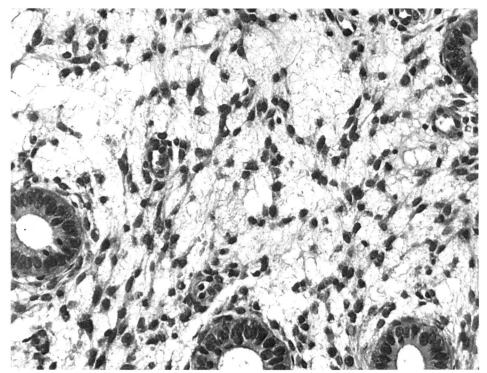

Fig. 60. Pathologic edema. H & E,×250.

Lymphatic cysts

(Figs. 61 and 62). Large lymphatic cysts lined by flat endothelium can be seen in the lower parts of the functional layer, occasionally surrounded by smaller cysts and patchy, focal or diffuse stromal edema. The lymphatic cysts can be differentiated from cystically dilated glands by their very flat endothelial lining.

Clinical correlation: These cysts develop in the same manner as focal or diffuse stromal edema and occasionally together with them. When blood vessels are ligated during hysterectomy, lymphatic channels may be blocked and become cystically dilated before the operation is finished.

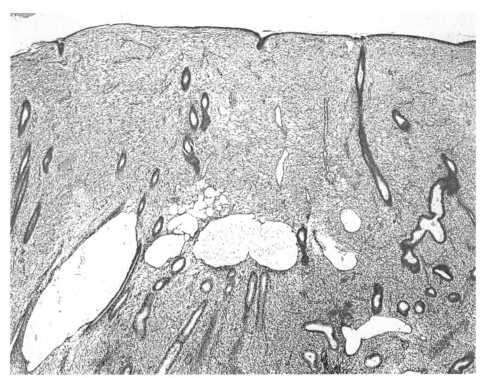

Fig. 61. Lymphatic cysts. H & E, ×25.

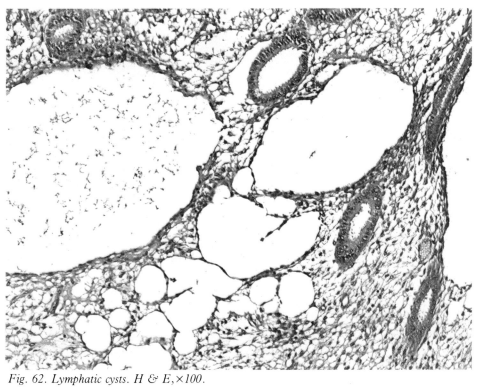

Fig. 62. Lymphatic cysts. H & E, ×100.

Apoplexia uteri

(Figs. 63, 64 and 65). Histologically a diffuse extravasation of blood throughout the superficial endometrial stroma is usually seen. The hemorrhage is confined to the upper layer of the endometrium and ends sharply at the internal uterine os. In less recent hemorrhages there may be necrosis of stromal cells and loss of reticulin fibers as well as degeneration of the glandular epithelium within the affected parts, and, rarely, scattered aggregates of polymorphonuclear leukocytes. The endometrium is usually atrophic and reactive changes remain restricted; therefore, hemosiderin-laden macrophages are not seen.

Morphologic differential diagnosis: The apoplexia must be differentiated from vascular thrombosis associated with tissue necrosis, which develops in a glandular cystic hyperplasia or after estrogen therapy.

Clinical possibilities and differential diagnosis: a) Chronic passive hyperemia with hemorrhages due to local mechanical obstruction of vessels by pressure from fibromyomas. b) Generalized reduced blood flow as in cardiac failure (Daly and Balogh 1968). c) Agonal or intraoperative hemorrhage by impaired circulation.

Distinction is possible according to the criteria for edema, but of negligible clinical importance.

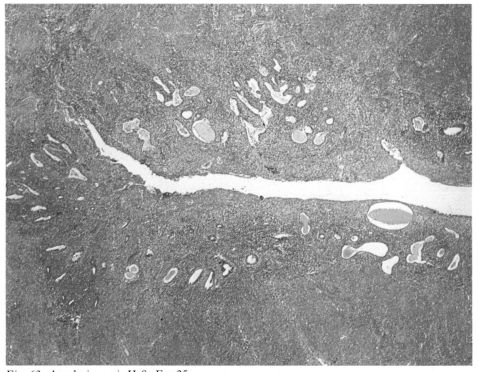

Fig. 63. Apoplexia uteri. H & E,×25.

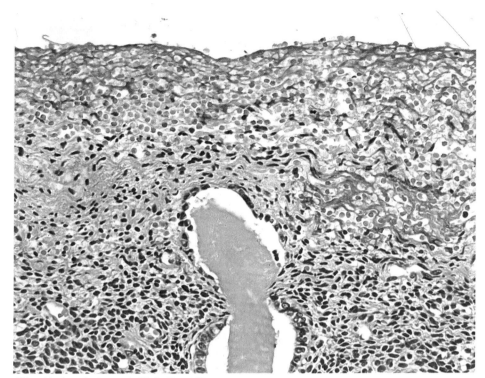

Fig. 64. Apoplexia uteri. H & E, ×250.

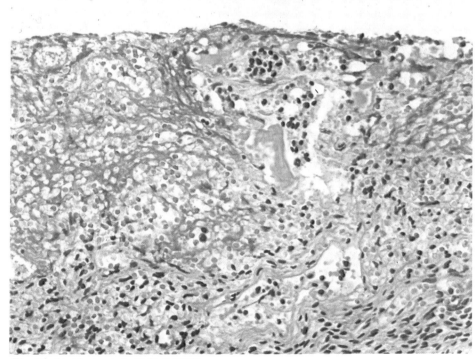

Fig. 65. Apoplexia uteri. H & E, ×250.

CHAPTER 4

Functional disturbances

If one follows the various stages of follicular maturation before and after ovulation, the arrest or persistence of this maturation can be divided into anovulatory and ovulatory disturbances of the endometrial function.

Anovulatory disturbances

During the reproductive period, the polycystic ovary syndrome is the most important cause of anovulation. Regardless of age non-functioning ovaries or deficient or prolonged follicular stimulation by a central or ovarian defect may cause an anovulatory disturbance (see Table 2, p. 112). Histologically, all resting or prolifera-tive stages from atrophy to hyperplasia may be found.

Diffuse atrophy

(Figs. 66, 67 and 68). The endometrium is very low and consists mainly of small spindle-shaped stromal cells covered by a cuboidal surface epithelium. Only occasional basal glands are found. Most of these are narrow and lined by low cuboidal epithelial cells with small, round nuclei with dense chromatin. Mitoses are lacking. The cytoplasm is scanty. Spiral arterioles are undeveloped. The extent of atrophy with total or subtotal loss of glands and more or less complete absence of enzymes and glycoproteins

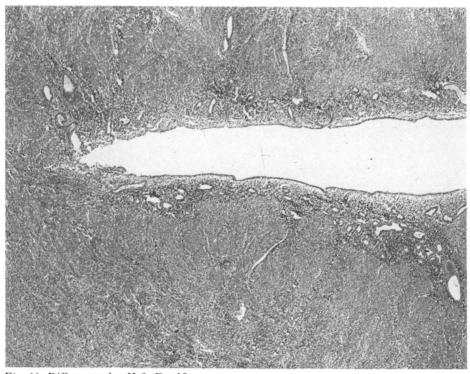

Fig. 66. Diffuse atrophy. H & E, ×25.

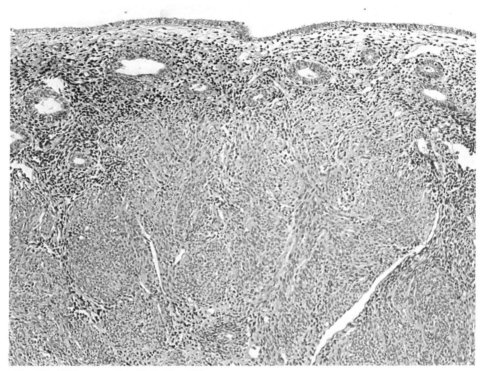

Fig. 67. Diffuse atrophy, H & E,×100.

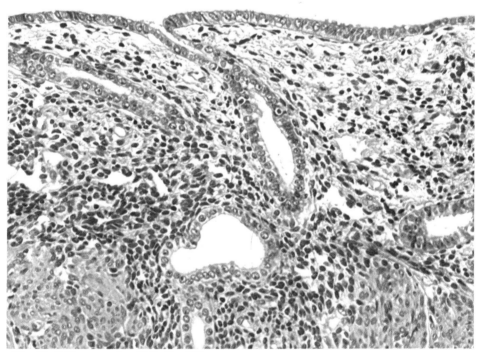

Fig. 68. Diffuse atrophy. H & E,×250.

is a measure of the severity and duration of the underlying change (Goldberg and Jones 1956; McKay et al. 1956; Lewin 1961; Gross 1964).

Clinical possibilities and differential diagnosis: a) Non-functioning ovaries i) before puberty and in the postmenopause, ii) due to a central or ovarian defect. b) Refractive endometrium. c) Iatrogenic suppression by gestagens (as with longstanding use of oral contraceptives or high dose gestagen-therapy).

Distinction is possible when the histologic diagnosis is correlated with the clinical history, age of patient, hormone therapy, and basal body temperature curve.

Focal pressure atrophy (Fig. 69) shows the same features as diffuse atrophy, but is localized, either overlying or facing a submucosal leiomyoma, whereas the surrounding endometrium may be quite different. Hence, if atrophy in curettings is only focal, its cause is mechanical rather than functional.

Resting endometrium

(Figs. 70 and 71). Resting endometrium has more glands than atrophic endometrium. Most of the glands are narrow, straight, and lined by a single row of columnar epithelial cells with chromatin-rich oval nuclei lying close together. The cytoplasm is scanty. The stromal cells are spindle-shaped and densely packed with very little edema focally. Mitoses are rare in glandular and stromal cells. Both cells contain only little RNA and their enzyme activities are low. The maximum height of the resting endometrium is 3 mm.

Clinical possibilities and differential diagnosis: a) Ovarian hypofunction shortly before puberty or regression in the early postmenopausal period. b) Hypoplastic ovary with very low estrogen production. c) Recent arrest of ovarian function (transitional stage to atrophy). d) Iatrogenic suppression by synthetic gestagens.

Distinction as in atrophy (see above).

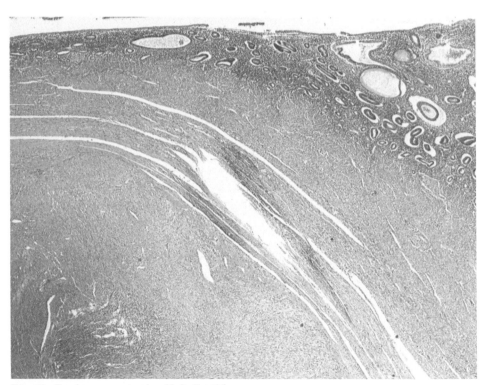

Fig. 69. Focal pressure atrophy. H & E, ×25.

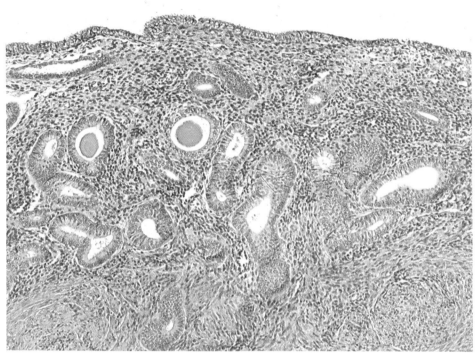

Fig. 70. Resting endometrium. H & E, ×100.

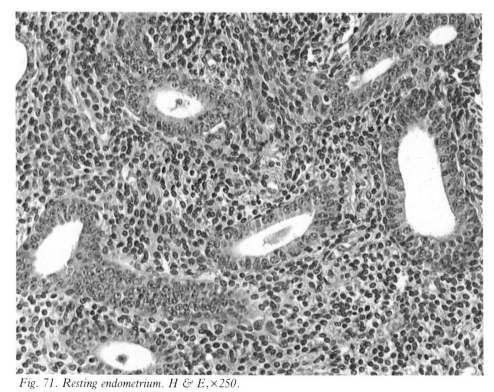

Fig. 71. Resting endometrium. H & E, ×250.

Deficient proliferation

(Figs. 72 and 73). The growth of the glands and stroma remains retarded as compared with that of the normal proliferative phase. The height of the endometrium is moderate, and the glands are slender and straight. The glandular and stromal cells are small. There may be focal variations in the degree of deficiency. Proliferation, protein synthesis and enzyme activities are reduced, but edema is usually present and more conspicuous than in the resting endometrium. There are only a few mitoses.

Clinical possibilities and differential diagnosis: a) Deficient follicular stimulation (central or ovarian defect: i) causing an anovulatory cycle, ii) as precursor stage of a deficient secretion). b) Iatrogenic suppression by hormone therapy (oral contraceptives).

Distinction as in atrophy (see p. 68).

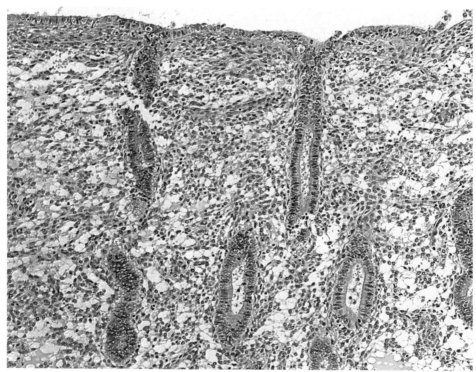

Fig. 72. Deficient proliferation. H & E, ×100.

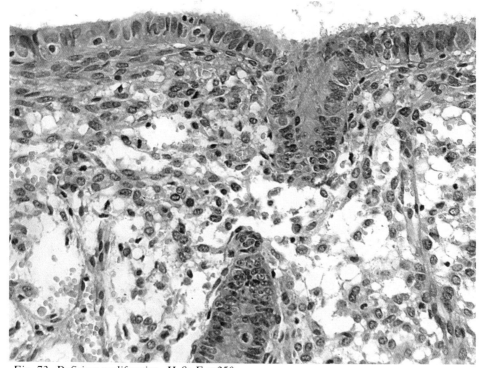

Fig. 73. Deficient proliferation. H & E, ×250.

Irregular proliferation

(Figs. 74 and 75). Here the growth of glands and stroma exceeds that of the normal proliferative phase. The endometrial glands are irregular in their shape, width and distribution, the lining epithelial cells are pseudostratified and form a dense row, their nuclei are large, rich in chromatin, and mitoses are frequent. The stroma is densely cellular and focally edematous. The height of the mucosa varies, but is in general considerable. The nuclear and cytoplasmic contents of DNA, RNA and enzymes are high.

Irregular proliferation is a transitional form to glandular cystic hyperplasia.

Clinical possibilities and differential diagnosis: a) Excessive estrogen production from: i) a persistent follicle, ii) polycystic ovaries with repeated anovulatory cycles, stromal hyperplasia or ovarian tumors. b) Absence of progesterone receptors in endometrium. c) Iatrogenic stimulation by synthetic estrogens.

Distinction as in atrophy (see p. 68).

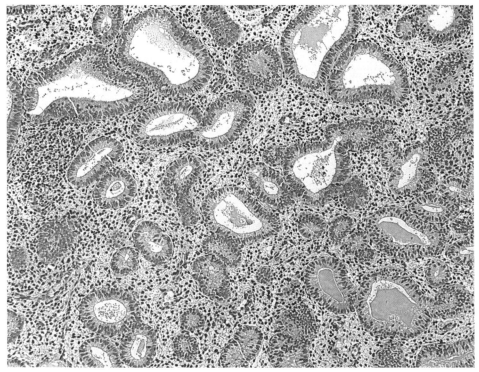

Fig. 74. Irregular proliferation without signs of secretion. H & E, ×100.

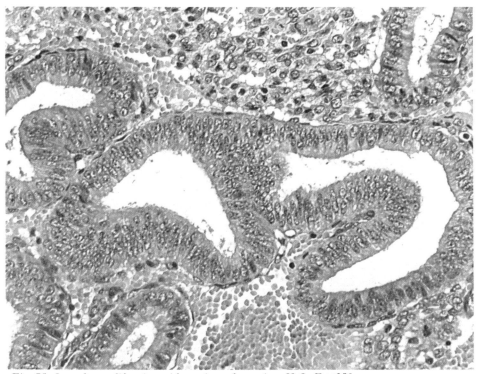

Fig. 75. Irregular proliferation without signs of secretion. H & E, ×250.

Deficient or irregular proliferation with focal abortive seretion (Figs. 76 and 77). The endometrial glands are either straight and narrow as in deficient proliferation, or vary in their width and distribution as in irregular proliferation, but the glandular epithelium is low with small, rounded, chromatin-dense nuclei. The scanty cytoplasm contains small amounts of glycogen, often in the shape of minute, basal or apical, vacuoles. The stroma corresponds to that in deficient or irregular proliferation and remains unchanged during the abortive secretion, which should not be misinterpreted as a sign that ovulation has taken place.

Morphologic differential diagnosis: Abortive secretion must be differentiated from late ovulation followed by absolute or relative corpus luteum insufficiency (refer to deficient secretory phase, p. 110). Except for severe corpus luteum insufficiency, this distinction is possible by judging (or measuring) the size of glandular nuclei and vacuoles, both of which are considerably smaller in non-ovulatory abortive secretion.

Clinical possibilities and differential diagnosis: a) Focal incomplete luteinization within a deficient or persistent follicle, when the LH peak does not suffice to induce ovulation. b) Use of oral contraceptives with suppression of ovulation as well as proliferation and secretory transformation.

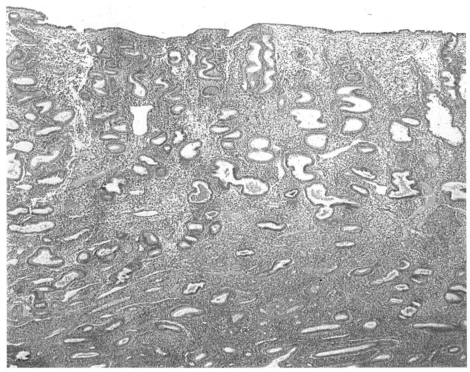

Fig. 76. Irregular proliferation with focal abortive secretion. H & E,×25.

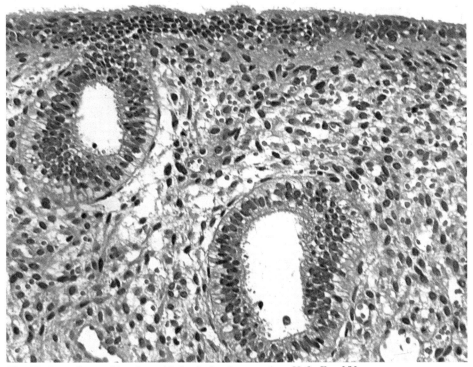

Fig. 77. Irregular proliferation with focal abortive secretion. H & E,×250.

Anovulatory withdrawal bleeding

(Figs. 78 and 79). In contrast to normal menstrual shedding, the anovulatory bleeding sets in without dissolution of reticulin fibers. In the early stages patchy edema and vascular thrombosis can be seen, resulting in hemorrhagic infarction and necrosis. Fresh hemorrhages can be demonstrated around deficiently or irregularly proliferating glands. In the advanced stages, fragments of tissue are shed but not dissolved properly because of the abnormal hormonal situation caused by lack of progesterone-withdrawal and relaxin secretion.

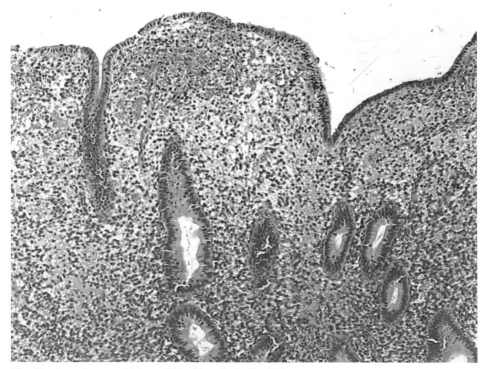

Fig. 78. Anovulatory withdrawal bleeding. H & E, ×100.

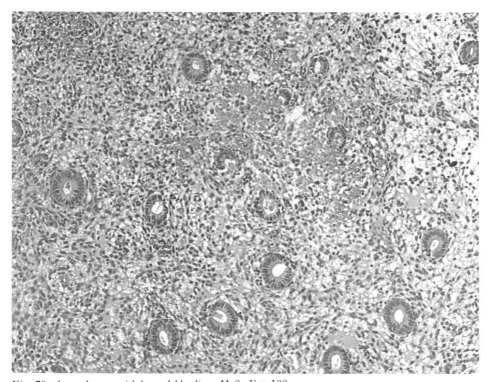

Fig. 79. Anovulatory withdrawal bleeding. H & E, ×100.

Glandular cystic hyperplasia

(Figs. 80-93). According to the extent of proliferative activity most or all of the endometrial glands are more or less cystically dilated and lined by pseudostratified, highly proliferating epithelium with enlarged, elongated, chromatin-rich nuclei in scanty, basophilic cytoplasm rich in RNA. Mitoses are frequent and often blocked in prophase or metaphase, which may explain the occurrence of clear cells within the glandular epithelium (Fuchs 1959) (see p. 56). The increase in activity of alkaline phosphatase is directly proportional to the level of estrogen (Filippe and Dawson 1968). The stromal cells are undifferentiated, densely arranged, and contain chromatin-rich nuclei in a sparse cytoplasm. Spiral arterioles are poorly developed. In contrast, the superficial capillaries and venules are numerous, dilated and often congested or thrombosed, resulting in areas of necrosis. The ground substance is partly depolymerized, containing mucopolysaccharides and often a fibrinous exudate (Schmidt-Matthiesen 1965) or hyaline thrombi.

In **slight glandular cystic hyperplasia** (Figs. 80, 81 and 82): the tall columnar glandular epithelium may still form a single row (Fig. 82).

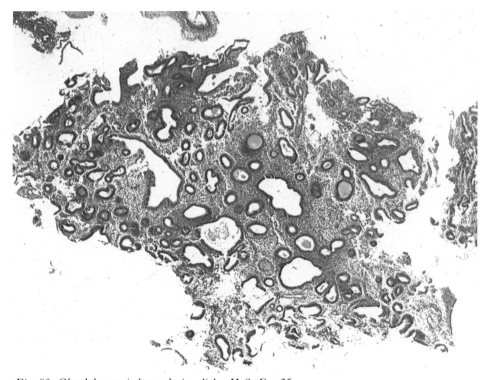

Fig. 80. Glandular cystic hyperplasia, slight. H & E, ×25.

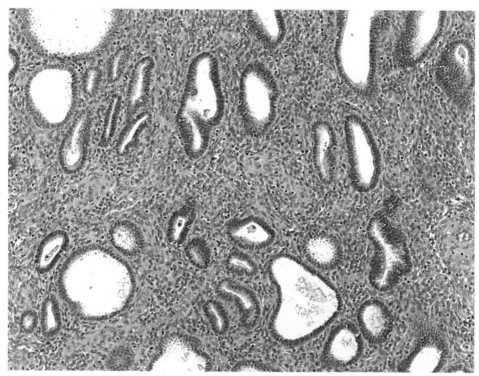

Fig. 81. Glandular cystic hyperplasia, slight. H & E,×100.

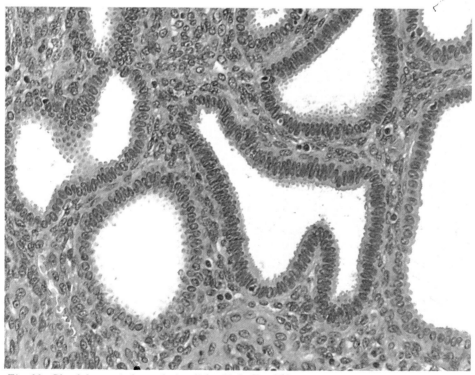

Fig. 82. Glandular cystic hyperplasie, slight. H & E,×250.

Severe glandular cystic hyperplasia (Figs. 83, 84 and 85), however, is always accompanied by an increase in glandular crowding (Fig. 83) and pseudostratification of the glandular epithelium (Figs. 84 and 85).

Clinical possibilities and differential diagnosis: a) Long-standing follicular persistence or repeated anovulatory cycles as in polycystic ovary syndrome. b) Excessive endogenous estrogen production by: i) ovarian stromal hyperplasia, ii) granulosa-theca-cell tumors or other estrogen-producing ovarian tumors, iii) adrenal glands. c) Unopposed exogenous estrogen. Distinction of a-c is possible only when the histologic findings are correlated with the clinical history and symptoms (see p. 126).

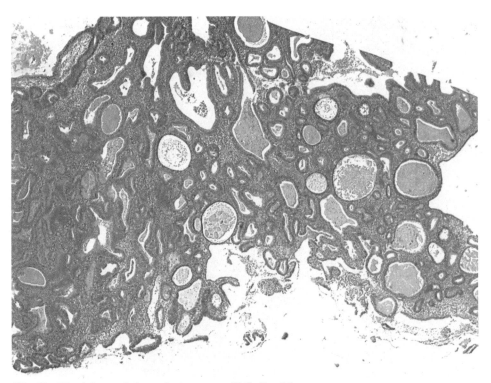

Fig. 83. Glandular cystic hyperplasia, severe. H & E, ×25.

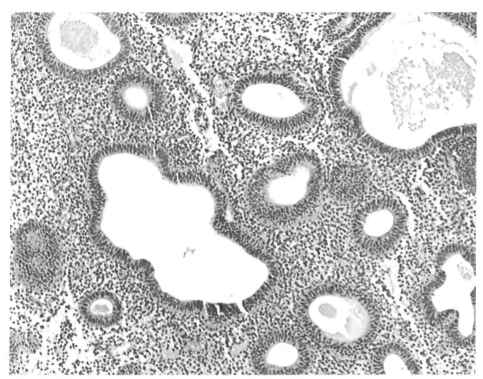

Fig. 84. Glandular cystic hyperplasia, severe. H & E, ×100.

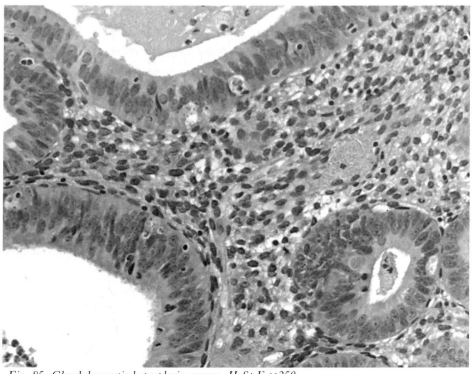

Fig. 85. Glandular cystic hyperplasia, severe. H & E, ×250.

Secretory transformation in glandular cystic hyperplasia (Figs. 86, 87 and 88) may occur in some or in most of the glands and is occasionally accompanied by various degrees of stromal differentiation. The glandular epithelium becomes single-layered again by intraluminal folding as in normally secreting endometrium, yet the nuclei remain small as in abortive secretion, and basal vacuoles are rarely seen (Fig. 87). The stroma may become predecidual or even decidual and may contain abundant endometrial granulocytes (Fig. 88).

Clinical possibilities: Secretory transformation may develop by: a) Sporadic luteinization in a persistent follicle. b) Exogenous gestagen therapy. c) Spontaneous ovulation (in the reproductive period).

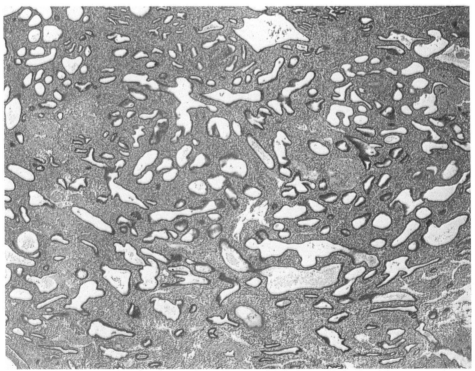

Fig. 86. Glandular cystic hyperplasia with secretory transformation. H & E, ×25.

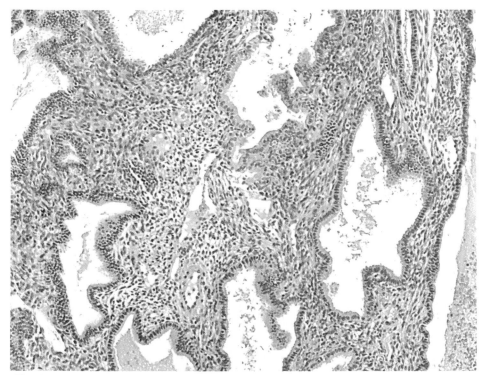

Fig. 87. Glandular cystic hyperplasia with secretory transformation. H & E,×100.

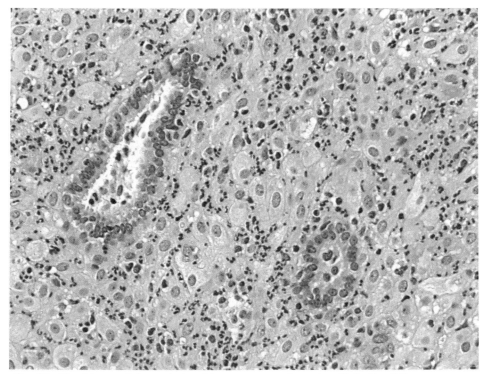

Fig. 88. Glandular cystic hyperplasia with secretory transformation. H & E,×250.

In **resting glandular cystic hyperplasia** (Figs. 89 and 90) the glands retain their cystic appearance but their lining epithelium becomes atrophic. Since the stromal cells also undergo shrinkage and atrophy, the cystic glands lie close to each other. DNA and RNA contents of glandular and stromal cells are greatly reduced. Mitoses are rare.

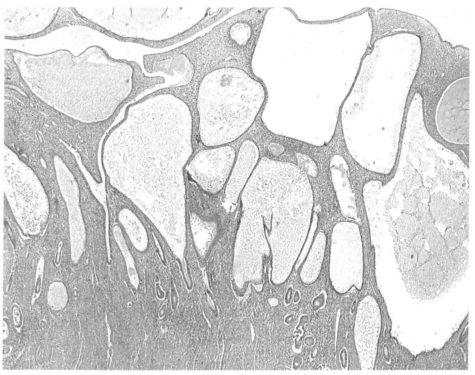

Fig. 89. Resting cystic hyperplasia. H & E, ×25.

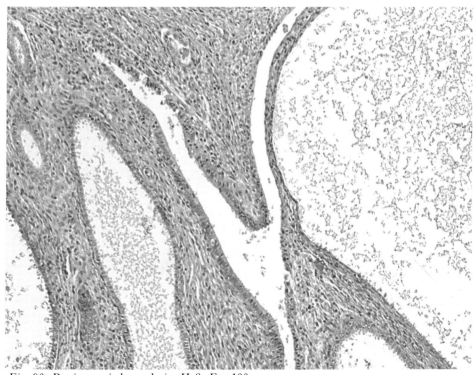

Fig. 90. Resting cystic hyperplasia. H & E, ×100.

Adaptation hyperplasia (Figs. 91, 92 and 93) may develop post partum or post abortum. Only some glands are cystically dilated; others are irregularly shaped and distributed. All glands are lined by highly proliferating epithelium, as in glandular cystic hyperplasia, and separated by a densely cellular stroma of large or shrunken, rounded cells. In the stroma there are characteristic patches of hyalinized decidual remnants surrounded by garland-shaped PAS-positive material (Figs. 92 and 93) and by chronic inflammatory infiltrates. In contrast to glandular cystic hyperplasia, spiral arterioles are still prominent. There are also fresh focal hemorrhages (Figs. 91 and 92).

Clinical possibilities: Adaptation hyperplasia is caused by post partum or post abortum persistence of follicles or by anovulation. The diagnosis is aided by recognizing decidual remnants or prominent spiral arterioles.

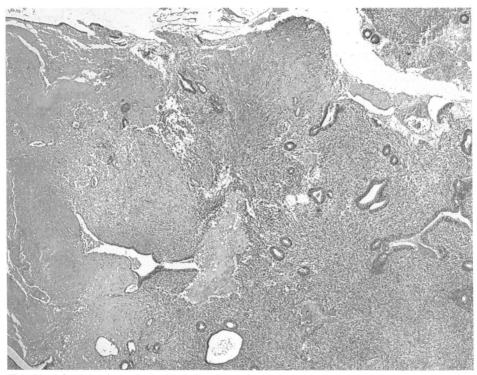

Fig. 91. Adaptation hyperplasia. H & E, ×25.

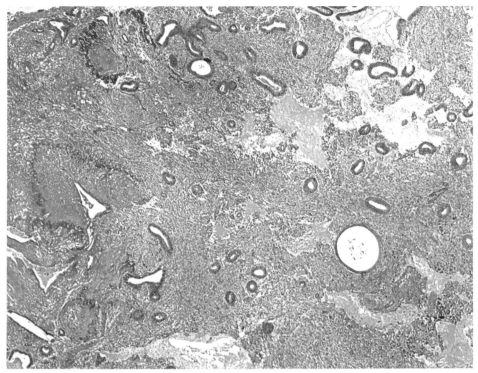

Fig. 92. Adaptation hyperplasia, PAS-reaction, ×25.

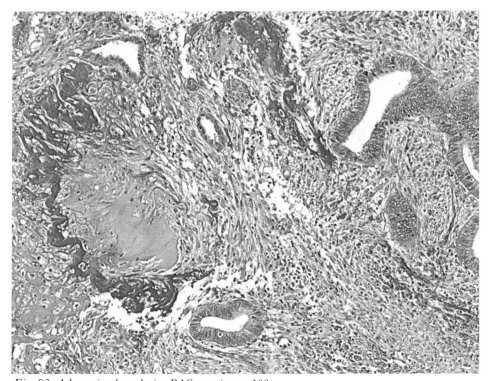

Fig. 93. Adaptation hyperlasia, PAS-reaction. ×100.

Adenomatous hyperplasia

(Figs. 94-107). Under the action of continuous unopposed estrogen the glandular proliferation progresses beyond the cystic dilation of glandular cystic hyperplasia by epithelial budding, branching and formation of new glands. The tall columnar glandular epithelium becomes pseudostratified or even stratified. In the elongated, enlarged, yet diploid, nuclei DNA synthesis and mitotic activity is greatly increased (Fettig 1965; Wagner et al. 1967). The sparse, undifferentiated cytoplasm accumulates abundant RNA. The stroma becomes rarefied.

In most instances it is possible to grade the adenomatous hyperplasia, although transitional forms do exist.

Mild (Grade I) adenomatous hyperplasia (Figs. 94, 95 and 96) may be focal or generalized. It is characterized by moderate glandular convolution, crowding, and pseudostratification of undifferentiated glandular epithelium. While some glands are still cystically dilated, others show beginning intraluminal infolding and budding. The spindle-celled stroma is preserved in some areas, but is focally quite sparse. The stromal cells are undifferentiated. Spiral arterioles are not prominent.

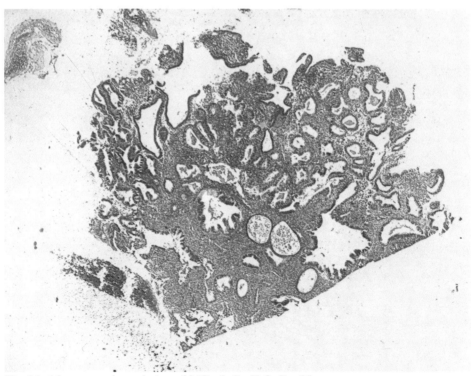

Fig. 94. Adenomatous hyperplasia, mild (Grade I). H & E, ×25.

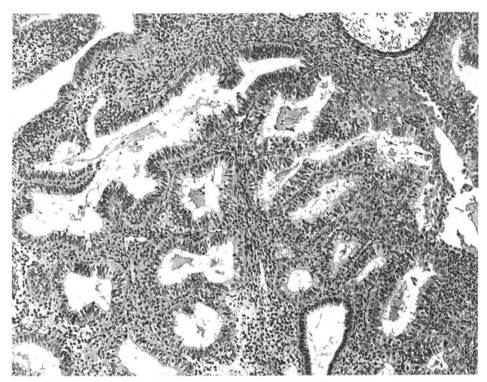

Fig. 95. Adenomatous hyperplasia, mild (Grade I). H & E, ×100.

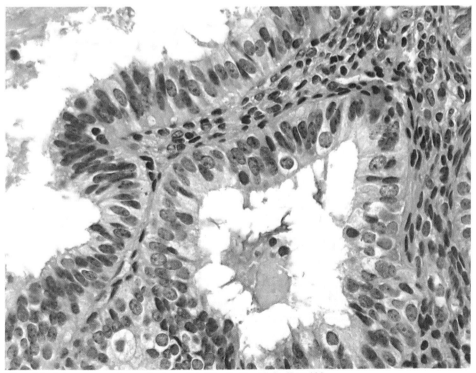

Fig. 96. Adenomatous hyperplasia, mild (Grade I). H & E, ×400.

Moderate (Grade II) adenomatous hyperplasia (syn. atypical hyperplasia) (Figs. 97, 98 and 99) shows diffuse and extensive adenomatous growth with focal early microalveolar formation, increased pseudostratification or stratification and intraluminal budding of glandular epithelium. The stroma is greatly reduced in some areas, resulting in a back-to-back position of the glands.

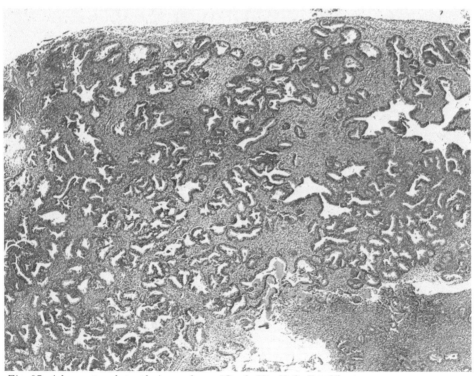

Fig. 97. Adenomatous hyperplasia, moderate (Grade II). H & E, ×25.

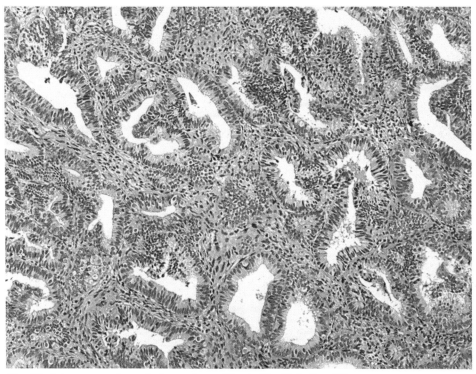

Fig. 98. Adenomatous hyperplasia, moderate (Grade II). H & E, ×100.

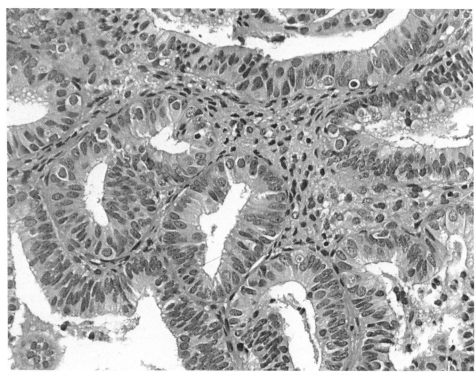

Fig. 99. Adenomatous hyperplasia, moderate (Grade II). H & E, ×250.

Severe (Grade III) adenomatous hyperplasia (Figs. 100, 101 and 102) meets all the criteria of Grade II adenomatous hyperplasia, and in addition, shows areas with atypical glandular epithelium: large, rounded, depolarized nuclei of various chromatin density are surrounded by pale eosinophilic cytoplasm with reduced amounts of RNA (MaKay et al. 1956).

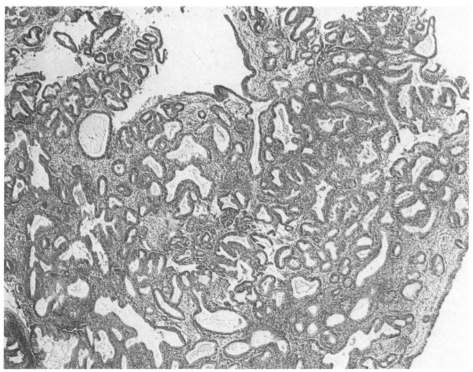

Fig. 100. Adenomatous hyperplasia, severe (Grade III). H & E, ×25.

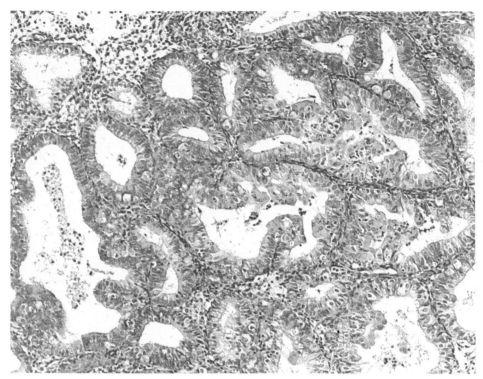

Fig. 101. Adenomatous hyperplasia, severe (Grade III). H & E,×100.

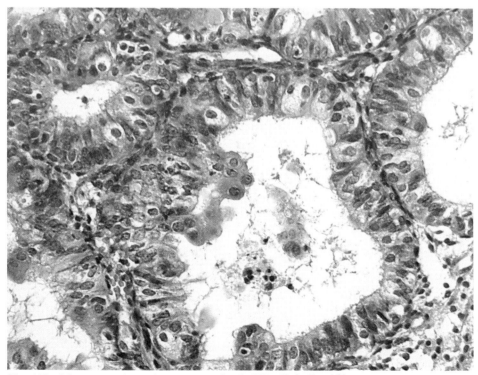

Fig. 102. Adenomatous hyperplasia, severe (Grade III). H & E,×250.

93

Special findings in adenomatous hyperplasia: Foci of *squamous metaplasia* (Fig. 103) that replace the glandular epithelium and fill the glandular lumina develop in some adenomatous hyperplasias as an individual reaction to the unopposed estrogen stimulation. The metaplastic cells contain regular nuclei in fairly abundant eosinophilic cytoplasm and are non-neoplastic. They are not fully matured, however, and are devoid of intercellular bridges. Mitoses are infrequent.

Groups of *foam cells* (Fig. 104) may be found in the stroma of over 50% of the adenomatous hyperplasias. They are of stromal origin (Fechner et al. 1979) and have stored lipids, which by their histochemical reactions are consistent with being cholesterol esters or estrogen derivatives (Dallenbach-Hellweg 1964; Dallenbach and Rudolph 1974). Their presence indicates high, unopposed estrogen levels. These cells are therefore useful in evaluating the prognosis of adenomatous hyperplasia: the higher their number, the poorer the prognosis. Foam cells also occur, but in a smaller percentage in glandular cystic hyperplasia, and they may persist in adenocarcinoma.

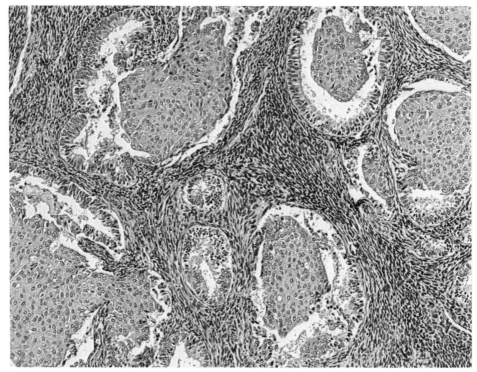

Fig. 103. Adenomatous hyperplasia with squamous metaplasia. H & E, ×100.

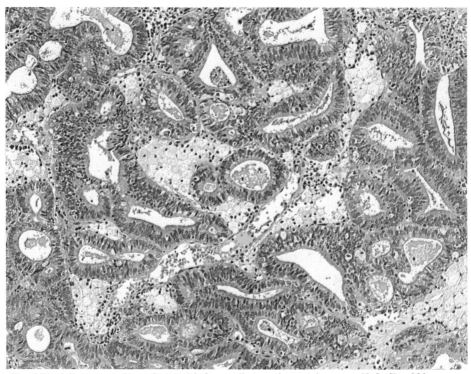

Fig. 104. Adenomatous hyperplasia with foam cells in endometrial stroma. H & E, ×100.

Juvenile adenomatous hyperplasia (Figs. 105, 106 and 107) represents a focal or diffuse severe type (of adenomatous hyperplasia) with depolarization and irregularity of glandular nuclei, frequent mitoses, pallor of the glandular cytoplasm, and complete loss of intervening stroma in large areas, giving rise to suspicion of invasive carcinoma. The lesion is limited to the endometrium (Fig. 105) and is considered non-invasive in women under the age of 40, since it can regress under progesterone stimulation (Dallenbach-Hellweg et al. 1971; Fechner and Kaufman 1974; Moukhtar et al. 1977).

Morphologic differential diagnosis of adenomatous hyperplasia: Adenomatous hyperplasia due to exogenous estrogen may be recognized by its focal distribution with considerable variation in morphologic appearance and by an excess of squamous metaplasia and foam cells. In Grade III adenomatous hyperplasia, areas of atypical glandular cells with depolarization of nuclei and pale cytoplasm must be differentiated from focal secretory changes within an adenomatous hyperplasia. Such a distinction is possible by noting the irregular arrangement of nuclei and the PAS reaction: the cytoplasm of Grade III adenomatous hyperplasia is PAS-negative, whereas the cytoplasm in secretory transformation is PAS-positive. Grade III adenomatous hyperplasia must, furthermore, be differentiated from early stromal invasion (see Fig. 194). The criteria for this distinction are listed under the discussion of early adenocarcinoma (see p. 168).

Clinical possibilities and differential diagnosis: a) Longstanding unopposed endogenous estrogen production, as in persistent anovulation (polycystic ovary syndrome), ovarian tumors, ovarian stromal hyperplasia, adrenals. b) Estrogen storage in fatty tissue. c) Impaired estrogen metabolism by liver damage. d) Longstanding estrogen therapy.

Distinction is possible by evaluating the clinical history.

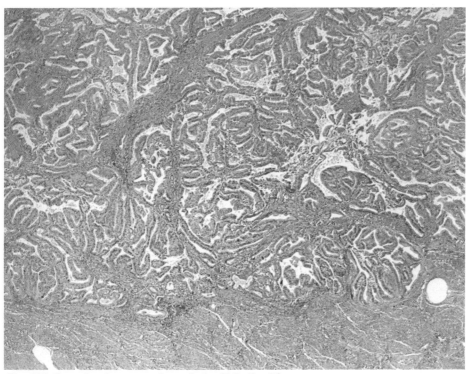

Fig. 105. Juvenile adenomatous hyperplasia. H & E, ×25.

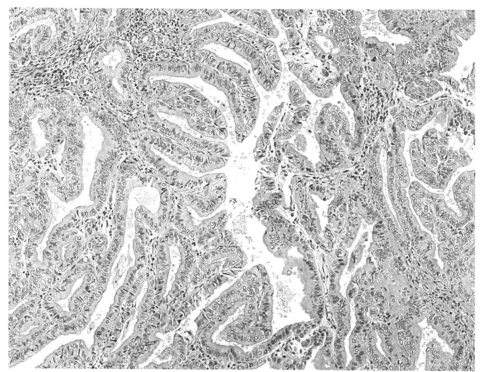

Fig. 106 Juvenile adenomatous hyperplasia. H & E,×100.

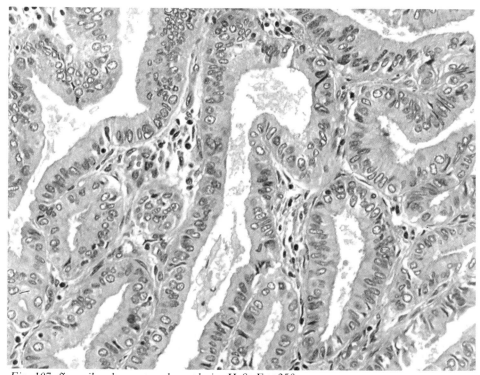

Fig. 107. Juvenile adenomatous hyperplasia. H & E,×250.

Adenomatous and stromal hyperplasia

(Figs. 108 and 109). In this condition the endometrial glands present the same appearance as in adenomatous hyperplasia. The endometrial stroma, however, rather than being rarefied is also hyperplastic. It consists of undifferentiated enlarged spindle-shaped densely distributed cells with oval nuclei rich in DNA and sparse cytoplasm rich in RNA. Mitoses are frequent in both glandular and stromal cells. Spiral arteriotes may be present (Fig. 109) but are not prominent (Hanson 1959).

Morphologic differential diagnosis: The combined adenomatous and stromal hyperplasia must be differentiated from a predecidual change of the stroma, as is occasionally observed under gestagen stimulation of an adenomatous hyperplasia, where the stromal cells are not undifferentiated but contain round nuclei and eosinophilic cytoplasm with low RNA content.

Clinical possibilities: Same as in adenomatous hyperplasia. The additional stromal hyperplasia is considered to be an individual variation due to the extensive stimulation by estrogen or its metabolic products.

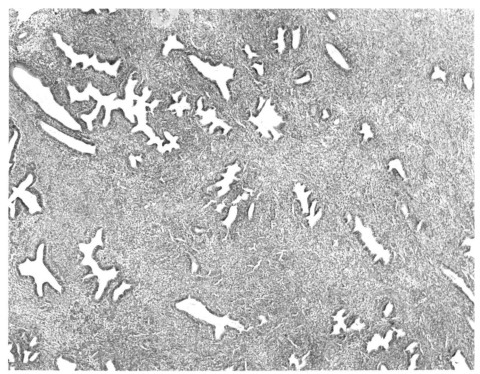

Fig. 108. Adenomatous and stromal hyperplasia. H & E, ×25.

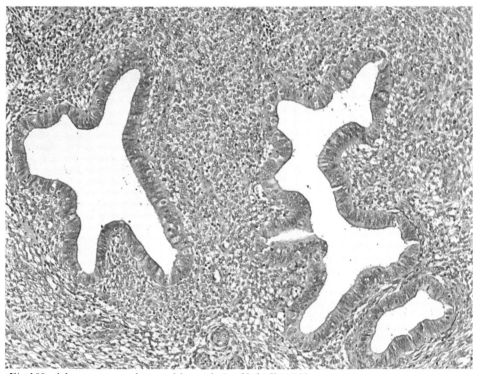

Fig.109. Adenomatous and stromal hyperplasia. H & E, ×100.

Focal hyperplasia

(Figs. 110 and 111). Focal hyperplasia differs from the diffuse form only by its limitation to one or a few areas of the endometrium which are usually located in the lower layers close to the basalis. Due to the growth pressure that develops, these foci become rounded, pushing the surrounding normal glands aside. In these regions glands and stroma are hyperplastic and undifferentiated. Noteworthy is the dense packing of stromal cells within the focus of hyperplasia (Fig. 111). Focal hyperplasias are not shed with menstruation, but are pushed upwards instead by the regenerating endomet-rium of subsequent cycles to become precursors of endometrial polyps.

Morphologic differential diagnosis: If isolated areas of focal hyperplasia are found in curet-tings, they must be differentiated from polyps: these are usually covered by surface epithelium, which is not present in focal hyperplasia.

Clinical possibilities and differential diag-nosis: a) Focal reactivity of endometrium to estrogens, while the surrounding endometrium has lost its estrogen receptor affinity. b) Focal loss of progesterone receptors with normal receptor content of surrounding endometrium.

Distinction is possible by observing the func-tional state of the surrounding endometrium.

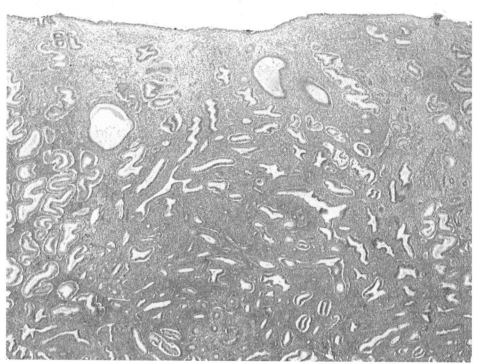

Fig. 110. Focal hyperplasia. H & E, ×25.

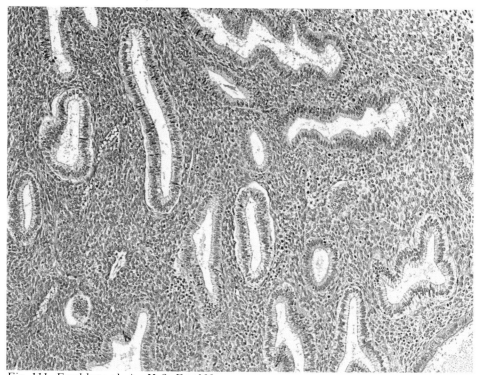

Fig. 111. Focal hyperplasia. H & E, ×100.

Basal hyperplasia

(Figs. 112 and 113). Basal hyperplasia shows the same structural features as focal hyperplasia. It may be diffuse (Fig. 112) or focal (Fig. 113). The diffuse form is the precursor of glandular cystic hyperplasia and may still be covered by normally proliferating or secreting endometrium which is pushed upwards. The focal variety is the precursor of endometrial polyps.

Clinical possibilites as in focal hyperplasia (see p. 100).

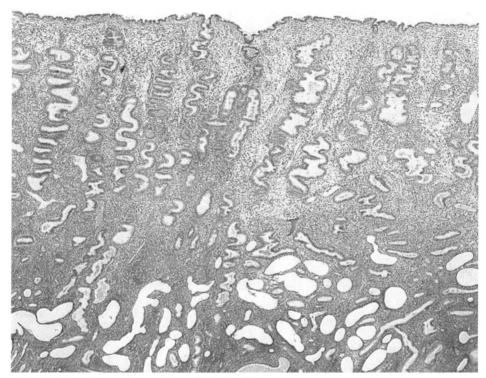

Fig. 112. Basal hyperplasia, diffuse. H & E,×25.

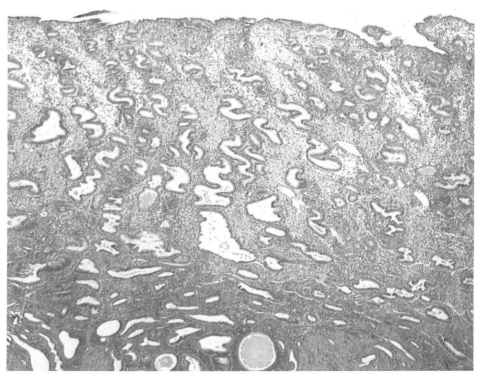

Fig. 113. Basal hyperplasia, focal. H & E,×25.

103

Endometrial polyps

(Figs. 114-118). Endometrial polyps develop from focal hyperplasias. At first a polyp has a broad base (Fig. 114). When the surrounding endometrium is repeatedly shed with menstruation, the base of the polyp becomes a slim stalk (Fig. 115). According to the structure of their glands we differentiate *glandular* (Figs. 114 and 116), *glandular-cystic* (Figs. 115 and 117), *adenomatous*, and *fibrous-cystic polyps* (Fig. 118). The glandular polyps resemble normal endometrium, but are recognizable by their being refractory to cyclic changes and by their fibrous stroma most clearly seen with the van Gieson stain (Figs. 116 and 118). The glandular-cystic and the adenomatous polyps differ from glandular-cystic and adenomatous hyperplasia only by their polypoid shape and their fibrous stroma. The fibrous polyps are regressive forms of glandular polyps and occur in old age. The glands that remain in them may be cystic or atrophic.

Morphologic differential diagnosis is necessary from papillary cystadenofibroma (see p. 198). Unless a connective tissue stain is used polyps or portions of them may not be recognized in curettings.

Clinical possibilities as in focal hyperplasia (see p. 100).

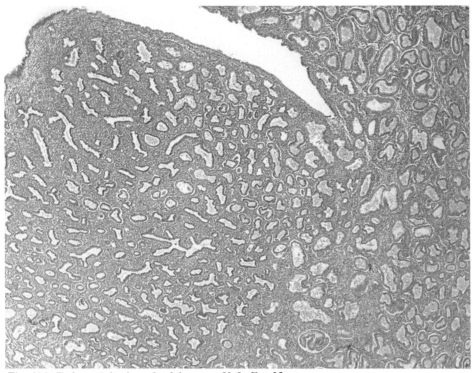

Fig. 114. Endometrial polyp, glandular type. H & E, ×25.

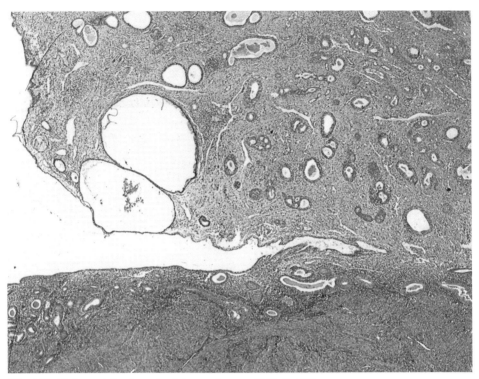

Fig. 115. Endometrial polyp, glandular cystic type. H & E,×25.

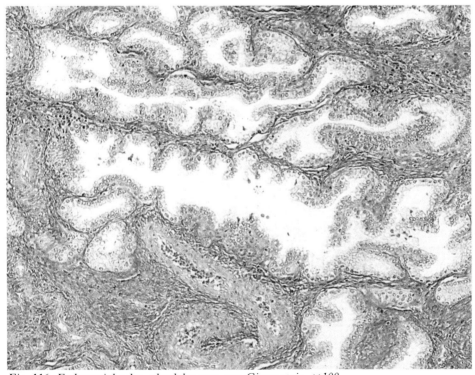

Fig. 116. Endometrial polyp, glandular type, van Gieson stain, ×100.

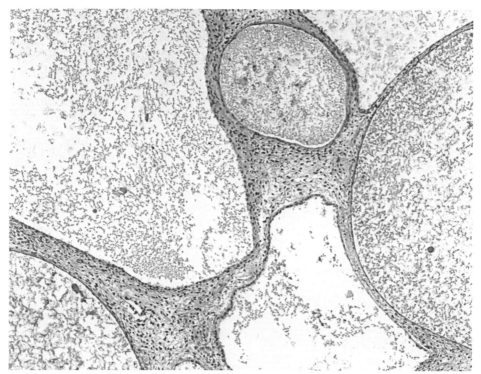

Fig. 117. Endometrial polyp, glandular cystic type, H & E,×100.

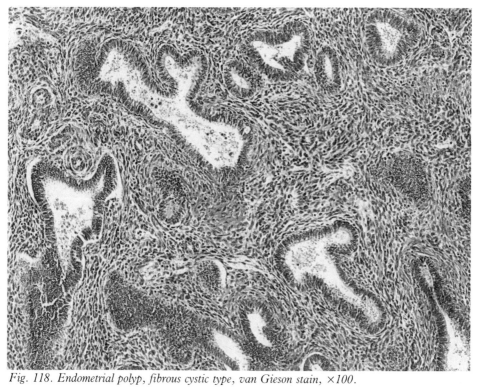

Fig. 118. Endometrial polyp, fibrous cystic type, van Gieson stain, ×100.

Ovulatory disturbances

Deficient secretory phase

This functional disturbance causes infertility and is usually associated with an insufficient corpus luteum. The deviation from normal function varies according to the degree of insufficiency, which may have central or ovarian causes. Since the result of treatment for this type of infertility depends on the accuracy of its diagnosis, a precise differentiation between the various patterns of the deficient secretory phase is of paramount importance (Gigon et al. 1970, Dallenbach-Hellweg 1984, see table 2, p. 112).

Deficient secretory phase with dissociated delay (Figs. 119, 120 and 121) This, the most frequent variety, shows unevenly spaced, poorly convoluted glands, a variation in the development of glands and stroma from region to region, and a dissociation of development between glands and their surrounding stroma.

This specimen has been taken on the 27th day of a menstrual cycle. Only very few glands even roughly correspond with the day of the cycle. Others are convoluted, lined by cells which either still contain elongated, chromatin-rich nuclei in a sparse cytoplasm, or which have rounded nuclei with occasional basal vacuoles remaining in their cytoplasm. The secretion in the glandular lumina may have just begun, or be advanced, or inspissated, and the lumina may also vary in their width. Some glands are straight, narrow and lined by undifferentiated proliferative epithelium. The stromal cells are either spindle-shaped and poorly differentiated or large and separated by focal edema. There are also occasional small hemorrhages. The spiral arterioles are small and underdeveloped. The general height of the endometrium varies slightly, the surface epithelium is tall columnar. The content of DNA, RNA, glycogen and mucopolysaccharides in glandular and stromal cells chiefly corresponds to the degree of differentiation, as compared with the normal cycle, and therefore also varies from area to area (Hughes et al., 1964; Ancla et al., 1967; Gore and Gordon, 1974).

Clinical possibilities: a) Deficient secretory phase due to ovarian insufficiency caused by an ovarian or central defect: inadequate luteinization and progesterone synthesis of granulosa cells or suppression of progesterone release by hyperprolactinemia. b) Deficient secretory phase caused by focal endometrial progesterone receptor defects. c) Irregular secretion caused by a climacteric disturbance in corpus luteum function.

Distinction can be made by exact statement of the day of the menstrual cycle and by determination of the plasma levels of FSH, LH and prolactin.

Deficient secretory phase with coordinated true delay: Since this entity is virtually identical with the beginning of a normal secretory phase, although the specimen was taken at the end of a menstrual cycle, the histologic diagnosis can only be made by knowing the exact day of the cycle. For histologic details we refer to Figs. 8 and 9, which could be a deficient secretory phase with coordinated true delay if taken not at the 16th but at the 26th, 27th or 28th day of the cycle. In occasional instances when the preceding proliferation is insufficient, the glands are small and narrow, the basal glycogen vacuoles barely reach normal size, and the stromal cells remain small and undifferentiated.

Clinical possibilities: a) Deficient secretory phase with coordinated true delay due to a central defect with inadequate stimulation of granulosa cells, or to an ovarian defect with impaired follicular development, or to a diffuse defect of endometrial progesterone receptor. b) Normal secretory phase on the 16th day of a menstrual cycle (2nd day after ovulation). c) Early structural changes following sequential therapy with oral contraceptives (see p. 142).

Distinction between a) and b) can be made by exact determination of the day of the menstrual cycle; the causes of the deficiency can be determined by measuring the plasma levels of FSH and LH.

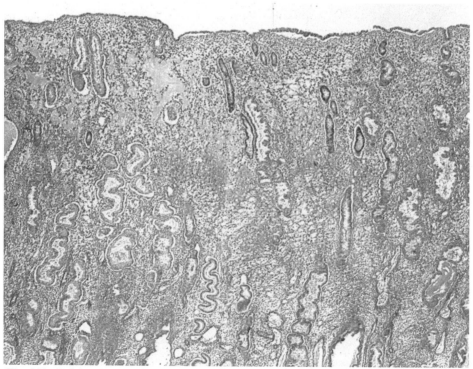

Fig. 119. Deficient secretory phase with dissociated delay. H & E, ×25.

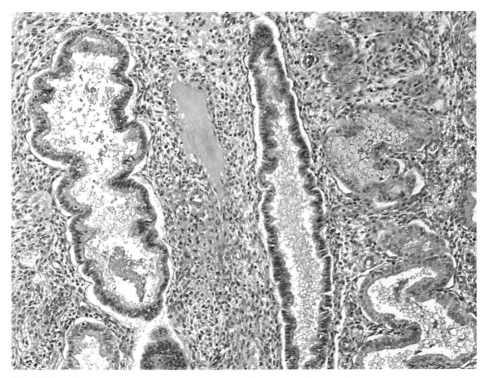

Fig. 120. Deficient secretory phase with dissociated delay. H & E, ×100.

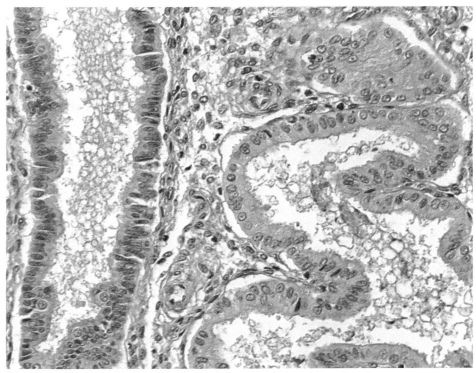

Fig. 121. Deficient secretory phase with dissociated delay. H & E, ×250.

Deficient secretory phase with coordinated apparent delay (Figs. 122, 123 and 124). The specimen was taken at the 27th day of a menstrual cycle. This functional disturbance is preceded by a persistent follicle with irregular proliferation of the endometrium and late ovulation: the secretory changes that are induced by ovulation are therefore only apparently delayed, not delayed in relation to the day of ovulation. The general height of the endometrium is considerable, but irregular. Part of the glands are cystically dilated, others narrow and only occasionally slightly convoluted. The glandular epithelium shows a beginning secretion with basal glycogen vacuoles and slightly rounded nuclei corresponding to the 2nd day after ovulation in a normal secretory phase. There is only slight variation in the size and extent of basal vacuoles, which are more pronounced in the glands not cystically dilated. The stroma cells are spindle-shaped or large and separated by focal edema. Spiral arterioles are present and only underdeveloped focally.

Clinical possibilities: a) Deficient secretory phase with coordinated apparent delay due to a central defect in LH stimulation, e.g. hyperprolactinemia with a delayed LH peak following follicular persistency with overproduction of estrogen. b) Irregular proliferation in the postmenopausal age period with sporadic luteinization of a follicular cyst, or following therapy with small amounts of gestagen.

Distinction can be made when the age of the patient, the menstrual history, and any given hormone therapy are known and, if necessary, by additional measurement of plasma levels of LH, FSH and prolactin.

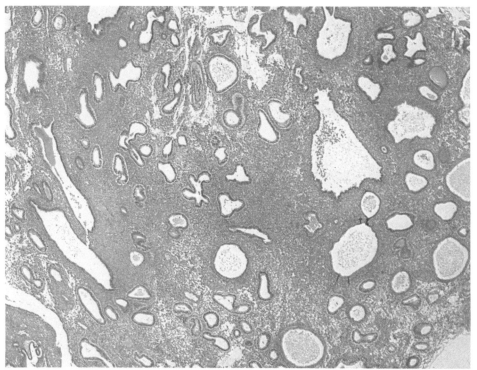

Fig. 122. Deficient secretory phase with coordinated apparent delay. H & E, ×25.

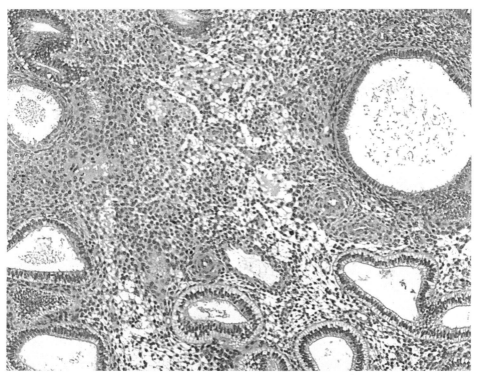

Fig. 123. Deficient secretory phase with coordinated apparent delay. H & E, ×100.

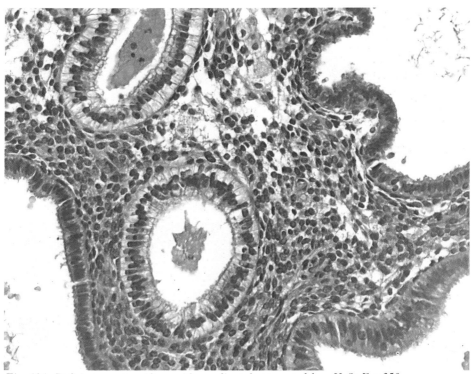

Fig. 124. Deficient secretory phase with coordinated apparent delay. H & E, ×250.

Table 2:

Functional disturbances of the endometrium in infertility

MORPHOLOGY:	POSSIBLE CAUSES:
Atrophy	a) Non-functioning ovaries (central or ovarian defect) b) Refractive endometrium
Deficient proliferation	a) Deficient follicular stimulation (central or ovarian defect) b) Anovulatory cycle
Irregular proliferation or hyperplasia	a) Persistent follicle b) Repeated anovulatory cycles (polycystic ovaries) c) Endometrium refractive to progesterone
Deficient secretory phase a) with coordinated delay b) with dissociated delay	a) Relative corpus luteum insufficiency due to high endogenous estrogen (apparent delay) or deficient estrogen priming (true delay) b) Insufficient corpus luteum (central or ovarian defect)
Abortive secretion	Non-ovulating, insufficient follicle with sporadic luteinization
Arrested secretion	Gestagen stimulation without ovulation, mostly exogenic
Asynchronous cycle	Disturbance of central regulation (direct or indirect by negative feedback mechanism)

Irregular shedding

(Figs. 125-134). In this condition the corpus luteum develops normally but fails to regress at the proper time and continues to secrete progesterone until this secretion subsides slowly and gradually. Consequently, endometrial regression is protracted and shedding is prolonged and irregular.

Early stage (Figs. 125-128): There are patchy foci of hemorrhagic dissociation (Fig. 125) and between these, preserved glands which have become star-shaped because of extensive shrinkage without disintegration (Figs. 126 and 127). The nuclei of the glandular epithelial cells are shrunken with dense chromatin, their cytoplasm is still fairly abundant and pale. The surrounding preserved stroma consists of densely packed, shrunken, yet rounded stromal cells and endometrial granulocytes still laden with relaxin granules. Consequently, the network of reticulin fibers remains intact (Fig. 128), preventing stromal and glandular dissociation (Dallenbach-Hellweg and Bornebusch 1970). The spiral arterioles show signs of slow regression and are often thrombosed, in part because of the prolonged bleeding.

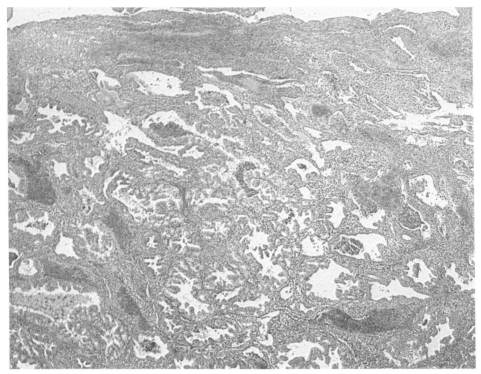

Fig. 125. Irregular shedding, early stage. H & E, ×25.

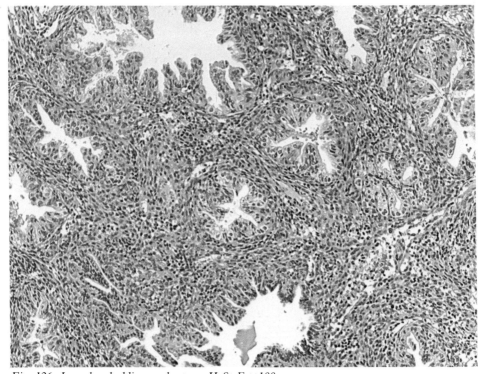

Fig. 126. Irregular shedding, early stage. H & E, ×100.

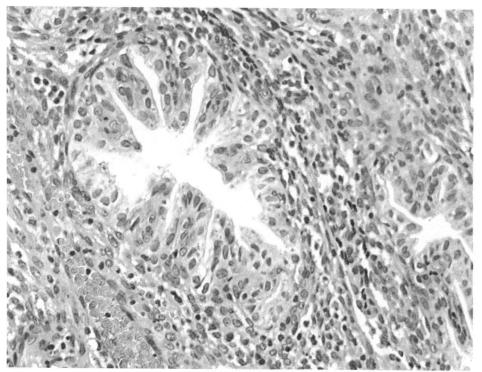

Fig. 127. Irregular shedding, early stage. H & E, ×250.

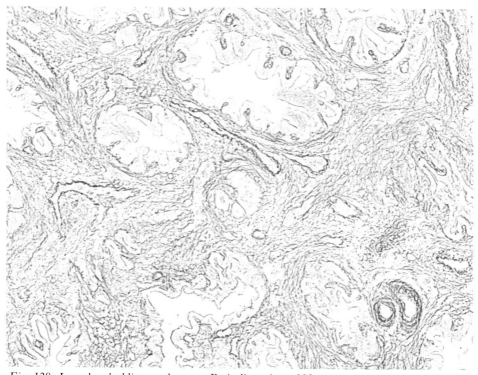

Fig. 128. Irregular shedding, early stage, Reticulin stain, ×100.

8*

Late stage (Figs. 129, 130 and 131): Larger regions of the endometrium are found to have undergone disintegration and hemorrhagic necrosis (Figs. 129). The intervening regions, however, are still intact. Their glands are further regressed, and their original star-shape is less pronounced but still apparent.

The nuclei of the lining epithelial cells are greatly shrunken and chromatin-dense, with sparse cytoplasm. Occasional deeper glands may already show regenerative or early proliferative changes, since they will become incorporated into the next cycle. The densely cellular stroma consists of small spindle-shaped cells (Figs. 130 and 131).

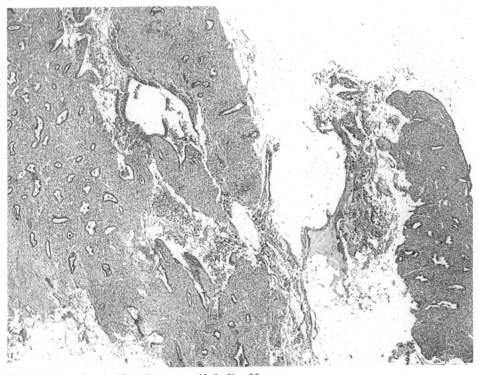

Fig. 129. Irregular shedding, late stage. H & E, ×25.

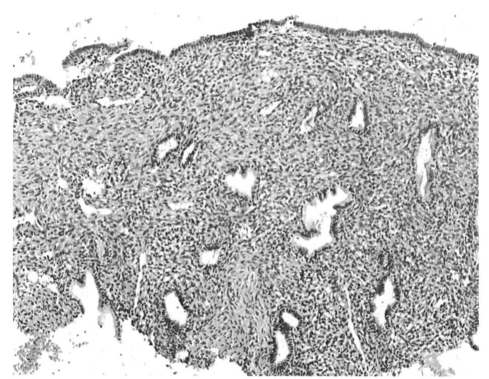

Fig. 130. Irregular shedding, late stage. H & E, ×100.

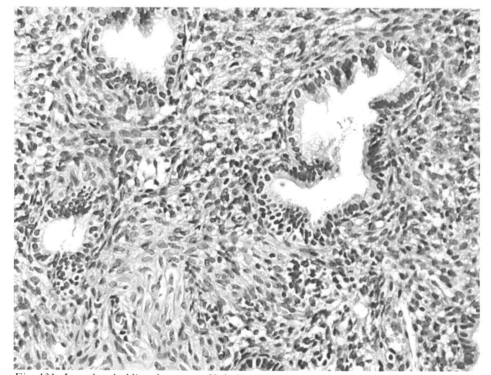

Fig. 131. Irregular shedding, late stage. H & E, ×250.

Arias-Stella-Phenomenon (Figs. 132, 133 and 134): In some instances the glandular epithelial cells have become greatly enlarged, yet with chromatin-dense and grotesquely shaped nuclei abnormally located in a very clear cytoplasm. This peculiar change (Arias-Stella 1954) is associated with high levels of gonadotropin produced by viable trophoblast (Figs. 133 and 134). There may be leukocytic infiltration of the stroma (Fig. 134) which does not react differently from that of irregular shedding without Arias-Stella-Phenomenon.

Histologic recognition and differential diagnosis of irregular shedding is not easy for the inexperienced. Characteristic is the diverse admixture of endometrial fragments in various stages of regression and dissociation. The condition must be distinguished morphologically from regressing glandular cystic hyperplasia with hemorrhage following secretory transformation: here part of the glands are still cystically dilated, and star-shaped glands are less conspicuous.

Clinical possibilities and differential diagnosis: a) Persistence of the corpus luteum by hyperstimulation from i) placental gonadotropin (in intra- or extrauterine pregnancy when the fetus has died, or with hydatidiform mole causing multiple corpus luteum cysts), ii) pituitary gonadotropin (during the first postpartum or post abortum menstruation, or in climacterium). b) Spontaneous polyovulation (Pepler and Fouche 1968). c) Gestagen therapy before the onset of or during the menses (Holmstrom and McLennan 1947).

Distinction is possible and of clinical importance particularly between irregular shedding due to hyperstimulation by placental remnants and that unassociated with previous pregnancy: a positive Arias-Stella-Phenomenon is always indicative of a recent intra- or extrauterine abortion, even when placental remnants cannot be found in the curettings. The presence of endometritis or hyalinized arterioles may help differentiate intra- from extrauterine pregnancy, whereas remnants of necrotic decidua may be found in both conditions. In the absence of previous pregnancy, precise clinical data are exceedingly valuable in the accurate interpretation of the underlying cause of irregular shedding.

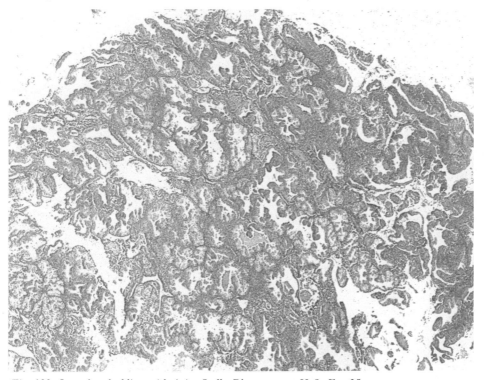

Fig. 132. Irregular shedding with Arias-Stella Phenomenon. H & E, ×25.

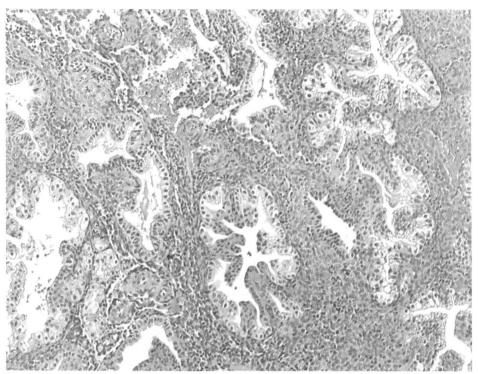

Fig. 133. Irregular shedding with Arias-Stella Phenomenon. H & E,×100.

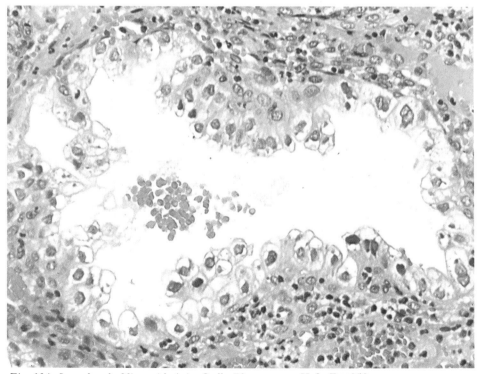

Fig. 134. Irregular shedding with Arias-Stella Phenomenon. H & E,×250.

119

Dysmenorrhea membranacea

(Figs. 135 and 136). The morphologic substrate for this clinical diagnosis is the finding of large, sheet-like pieces of more or less well-preserved predecidual or decidual endometrium which have been shed undissociated from the uterine cavity. The plane of separation is clearly recognized by the zone of hemorrhagic necrosis (Fig. 135). The endometrial glands are more or less convoluted, are lined by low cuboidal cells with round nuclei in a sparse cytoplasm. The glandular lumina may be narrow or wide but are usually devoid of secretion. The abundant endometrial stroma consists of predecidual or decidual cells (Fig. 136). Occasionally, inflammatory infiltrates extend beyond the line of demarcation.

Morphologic differential diagnosis: It may be difficult to distinguish between the dysmenorrhea membranacea that follows intra- or extrauterine abortion and that induced by a persistent corpus luteum unassociated with pregnancy when placental remnants or characteristics of an Arias-Stella-Phenomenon are lacking, since persistent progesterone stimulation may also transform the endometrial cells into decidual cells indistinguishable from those of a pregnancy (Spechter 1953).

Distinction is possible, however, when the endometrial glands are non-convoluted, narrow and lined by atrophic epithelium: such an "arrested secretion", which can also be shed in the shape of a decidual cast, is seen only after gestagen therapy (see Fig. 149).

Clinical interpretation and differential diagnosis: Same as for irregular shedding (p. 118). A decidual cast may be expelled in one piece when disintegration of reticulin fibers fails to occur in the absence of relaxin discharge from endometrial granulocytes. Relaxin is retained with persistent progesterone secretion or during gestagen therapy. Decidual casts may then be discharged when gestagen therapy is discontinued ("hormonal curettage").

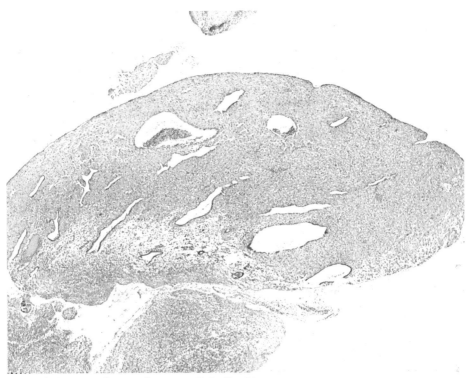

Fig. 135. Dysmenorrhea membranacea. H & E, ×25.

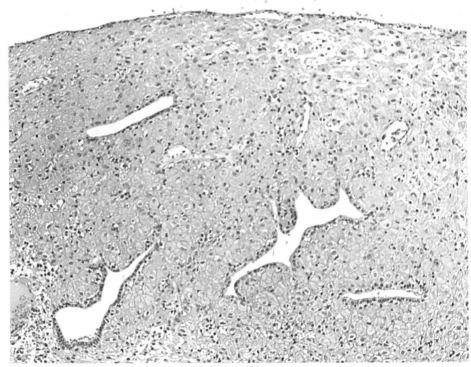

Fig.136. Dysmenorrhea membranacea. H & E, ×100.

Secretory hypertrophy

(Figs. 137-142). This condition is observed only in the preclimacteric period. The hypersecreting endometrium may measure 1 cm in height. Two types may be distinguished, but combinations of the two are also seen.

In the **glandular type** (Figs. 137, 138 and 139): Densely arranged convoluted hypersecreting glands occupy all layers of the endometrium up to the surface epithelium (Figs. 137 and 138). Their lining epithelial cells contain round nuclei in abundant, secreting, often clear cytoplasm, their serrated lumina are filled with secretion (Fig. 139). Between these large glands groups of slightly underdeveloped glands can be distinguished. The sparse stroma consists of densely arranged, large, rounded predecidual cells and endometrial granulocytes. Spiral arterioles are prominent.

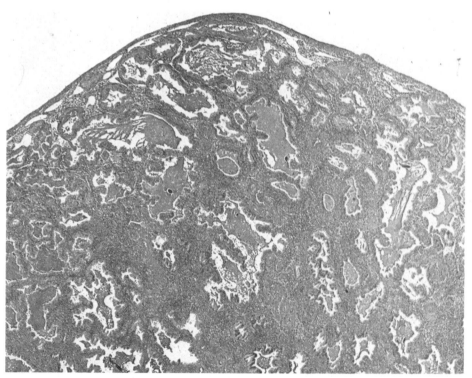

Fig. 137. Secretory hypertrophy, glandular type. H & E,×25.

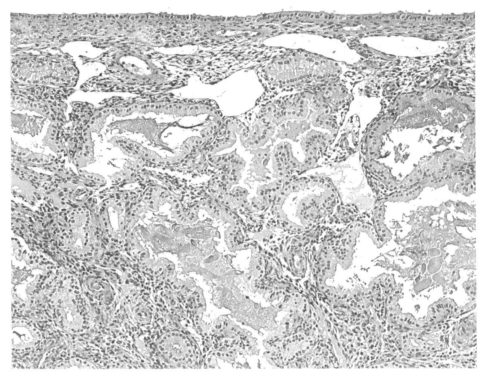

Fig. 138. Secretory hypertrophy, glandular type. H & E,×100.

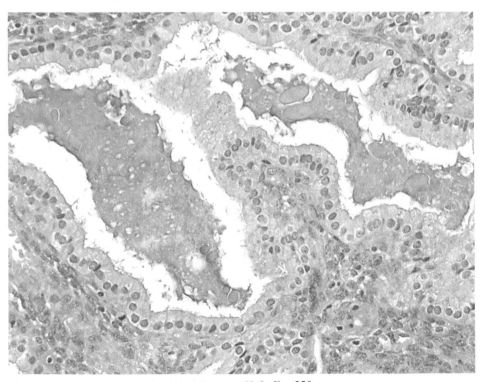

Fig. 139. Secretory hypertrophy, glandular type. H & E,×250.

In the **decidual type** (Figs. 140, 141 and 142): The endometrial glands appear very similar to those described above (Fig. 141), but are in scattered groups, widely separated by a well preserved compact stroma consisting of pre-decidual cells and endometrial granulocytes (Fig. 142). In contradistinction to premenstrual endometrium, the compact stroma is not limited to the upper layer of the endometrium but arranged in patches throughout all layers (Fig. 140). There may be focal stromal edema.

Morphologic differential diagnosis: Secretory hypertrophy must be differentiated from decidual transformation in early implantation of an intrauterine pregnancy or that accompanying an extrauterine pregnancy. The endometrial specimen must therefore be screened carefully for trophoblasts or early placental villi. A focal Arias-Stella-Phenomenon will also aid in the detection of a hypersecretion associated with pregnancy. In the absence of these signs, clinical data are needed in the differential diagnosis.

Clinical correlation: Climacteric hyperfunction of the corpus luteum, possibly through excessive production of pituitary gonadotropin.

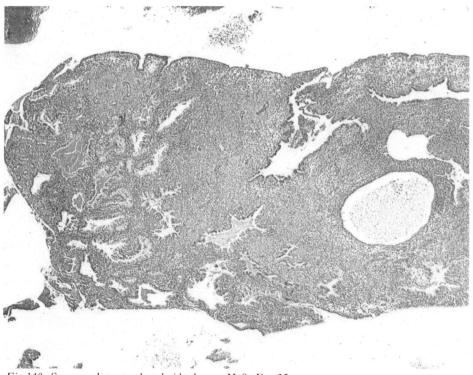

Fig.140. Secretory hypertrophy, decidual type. H & E, ×25.

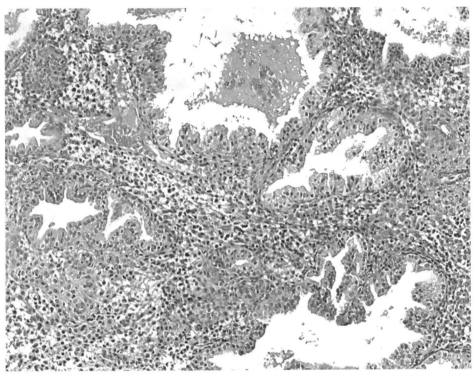

Fig. 141. Secretory hypertrophy, decidual type. H & E, ×100.

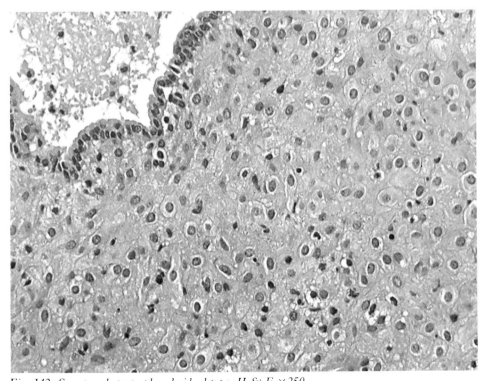

Fig. 142. Secretory hypertrophy, decidual type. H & E, ×250.

CHAPTER 5

Iatrogenic changes

After hormonal therapy

Most synthetic hormones are extremely potent, since the target cells they stimulate are exquisitely responsive even to low concentrations and react promptly with characteristic changes, which may differ from those induced by the natural hormones.

Estrogen-induced hyperplasia

(Figs. 143-147). In the reaction to synthetic estrogens, individual variations and the age of the patient must be taken into account (Hempel et al. 1977). With prolonged administration of small doses of estradiol (20-100 μg daily) various stages of endometrial hyperplasia develop.

In young women below 40 years of age (Figs. 143 and 144): The hyperplasia is often focal (Fig. 143), but within each focus the hyperplastic glands are evenly distributed and show an adenomatous growth with pseudostratification of the epithelial cells (Fig. 144). Their nuclei are elongated and chromatin-rich, occasionally slightly rounded when tiny vacuoles become visible in the cytoplasm, which is otherwise slightly eosinophilic. Nodules of squamous metaplasia may be numerous. The stroma is rarefied and in some regions absent. Mitoses are frequent in the glandular epithelium, whereas the stromal cells are inactive.

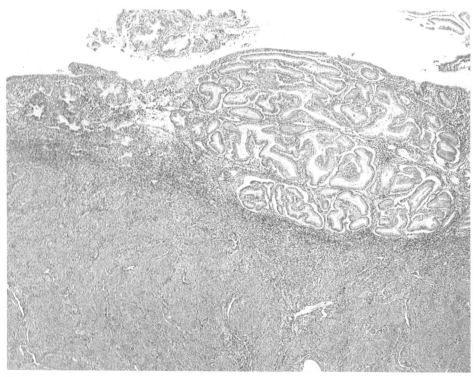

Fig. 143. Estrogen-induced hyperplasia in the young woman. H & E, ×25.

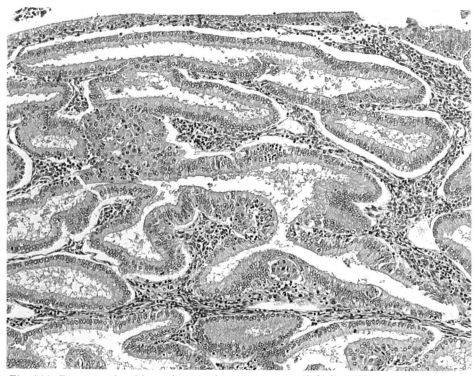

Fig. 144. Estrogen-induced hyperplasia in the young woman. H & E, ×100.

In old age (Figs 145, 146 and 147): Many endometrial glands are cystically dilated (Fig. 145). Their lining epithelium varies from gland to gland (Fig. 147): it may be pseudostratified or stratified. The nuclei are large, round or elongated, pale or chromatin-rich and depolarized. Mitoses are frequent. The glandular cytoplasm may be sparse and basophilic, eosinophilic, or clear when the whole cell appears swollen. The remaining stroma between the abundant glands is undifferentiated, dense or focally edematous and may contain groups of endometrial foam cells, which store estrogen metabolites. Spiral arterioles are very scanty or absent.

Morphologic differential diagnosis: In contrast to the hyperplasias caused by endogenous estrogen, those developing after estrogen therapy are often multicentric or polypoid, show great variation in structure from gland to gland and may contain numerous nodules of squamous metaplasia. Diffuse hyperplasia as caused by endogenous estrogen may, however, be seen, although much less frequently.

Clinical possibilities and differential diagnosis: a) Longstanding estrogen therapy. b) Endogenous hyperestrogenism.

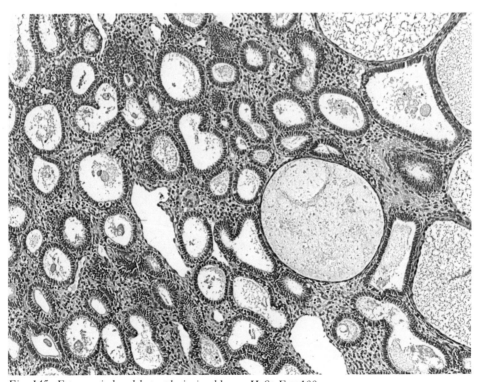

Fig. 145. Estrogen-induced hyperplasia in old age. H & E, ×100.

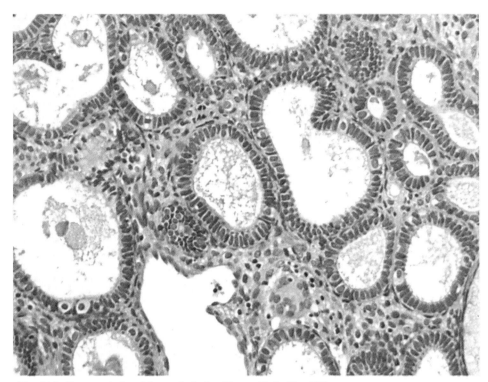

Fig. 146. Estrogen-induced hyperplasia in old age. H & E, ×250.

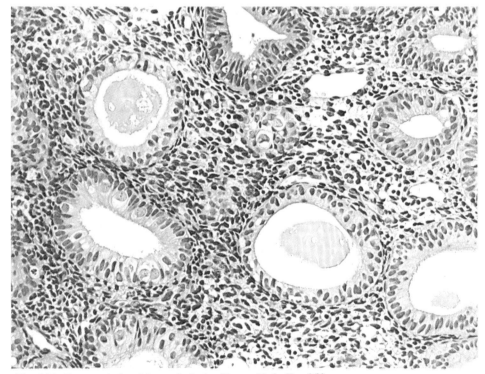

Fig. 147. Estrogen-induced hyperplasia in old age. H & E, ×250.

Gestagen induced regression

(Figs. 148-152). The synthetic gestagens differ both chemically and metabolically from natural progesterone. Because of their great potency, their action on the target cells is exaggerated. The intensity of the morphologic changes depends not only on the potency of the gestagen used but also on the dosis, length of administration and hormonal status of the patient.

Arrested secretion (Figs. 148 and 149): Develops after three months of gestagen therapy when a feedback mechanism has inhibited the secretion of FSH and thereby prevented proliferation of endometrial glands. Consequently, the glands are sparse, narrow, and lined by atrophic epithelium, whereas the stroma is decidualized and rich in endometrial granulocytes. The arrest in secretion is the result of the preceding suppression of proliferation, whereas the stroma still shows a very distinct gestagen effect.

Clinical correlation: Therapy with synthetic gestagens only (gestagen preparation alone or combined with low dose estrogen as oral contraceptives). There is no known endogenous disturbance which results in arrested secretion.

Fibrous atrophy (Fig. 150): Develops from arrested secretion when the gestagen therapy is continued for six months or longer: here the glands have completely disappeared, and the stroma consists merely of very few layers of small undifferentiated spindle cells. Only the surface epithelium is still distinctly proliferating.

Morphologic differential diagnosis: Atrophy from endogenous causes is seldom as complete as that following longstanding gestagen therapy; pressure atrophy is always focal (cf. Figs. 66-69).

Clinical possibilities and differential diagnosis: a) Longstanding therapy with synthetic gestagens. b) Complete arrest of ovarian function in old age or after bilateral ovariectomy. c) Endometrial refractoriness to hormones. d) Pressure atrophy.

Distinction is possible by evaluating the clinical history.

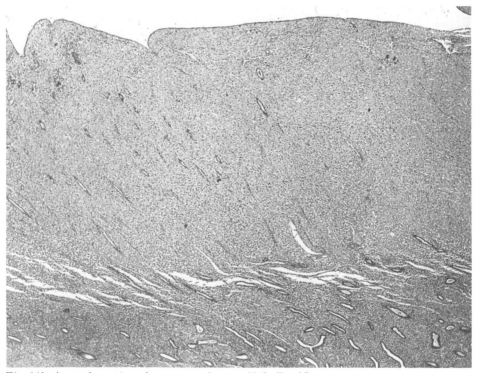

Fig. 148. Arrested secretion after gestagen therapy. H & E, ×25.

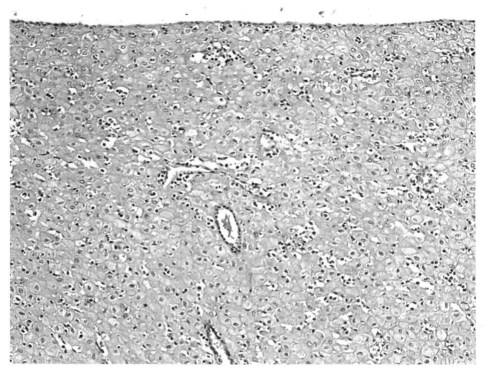

Fig. 149. Arrested secretion after gestagen therapy. H & E, ×100.

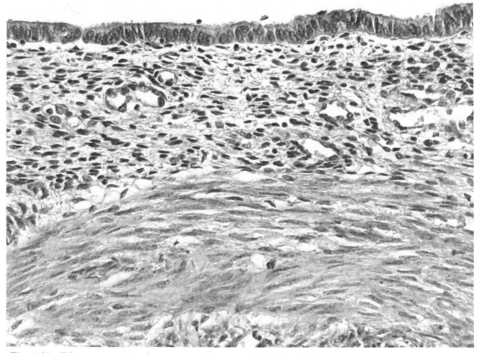

Fig. 150. Fibrous atrophy after gestagen therapy. H & E, ×250.

9*

Gestagen therapy of adenomatous hyperplasia or adenocarcinoma (Figs. 151 and 152): Results in more or less incomplete secretory transformation of the previously proliferating glandular epithelium. The nuclei become round, mitoses are inhibited (Nordqvist 1964), and the cytoplasm may show signs of early, advanced or abortive secretion (John et al. 1974), whereas the sparse stroma remains almost unchanged. Since considerably more endogenous estrogen has to be counteracted than in a normal cycle, the stage of arrested secretion will only be reached after gestagen therapy in very high doses (150 mg – 250 mg daily) for six to twelve months or even longer (Kistner 1959; Kistner et al. 1965; Eichner and Abellera 1971). Whereas adenomatous hyperplasia may disappear completely after longlasting high doses of gestagen, only a growth arrest can be achieved in invasive carcinoma.

Clinical possibilities and differential diagnosis: a) Gestagen therapy of adenomatous hyperplasia or adenocarcinoma. b) Endogenous production of progesterone, e.g. spontaneous ovulation in a young woman with adenomatous hyperplasia. c) Secretory type of adenocarcinoma (cf. Figs. 203-205).

Distinction is possible only by evaluation of the clinical history.

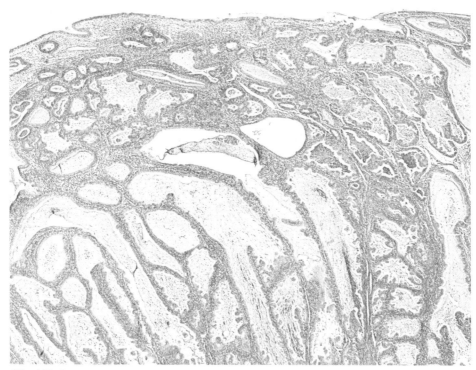

Fig. 151. Incomplete secretory transformation after gestagen therapy of adenomatous hyperplasia. H & E, ×25.

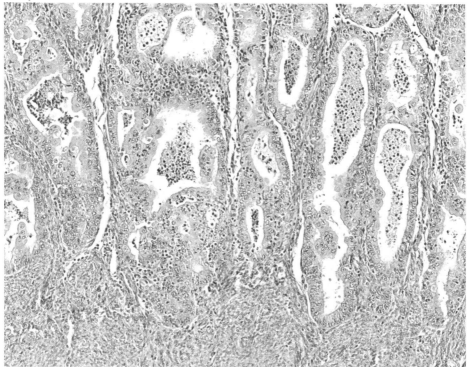

Fig. 152. Incomplete secretory transformation after gestagen therapy of adenomatous hyperplasia. H & E, ×100.

Combination therapy

(Figs. 153-165). The combined action of both hormones is the precise result of dose and potency of each hormone given and the level of endogenous hormones available for reaction. Oral contraceptives, as the most frequently used combined preparations, usually have a predominant gestagen effect, resulting in abortive secretion.

Abortive secretion (Figs. 153, 154 and 155): The endometrial glands are diminished in number, narrow, straight and lined by flat epithelium with small, round, chromatin-dense nuclei in sparse eosinophilic cytoplasm, only occasionally containing tiny vacuoles of glycogen not indicative of ovulation (Fig.. 155). Protein synthesis is reduced (Verhagen and Themann 1970; Toth et al. 1972). The stromal cells are mostly spindle-shaped, incompletely differentiated and separated by edema.

Clinical possibilities and differential diagnosis: a) Combined hormone therapy with predominance of gestagen as in most oral contraceptives. b) Sporadic luteinization in an insufficient follicle (cf. Figs. 76 and 77).

Distinction may be possible only by evaluating the clinical history.

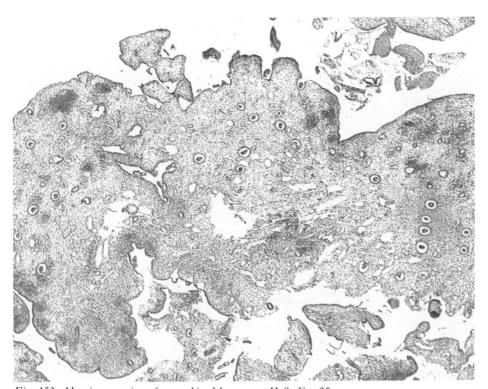

Fig. 153. Abortive secretion after combined hormones. H & E, ×25.

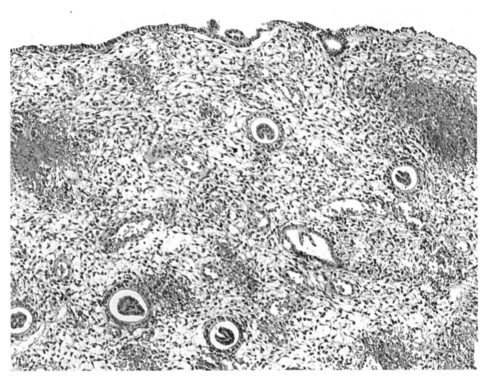

Fig. 154. Abortive secretion after combined hormones. H & E,×100.

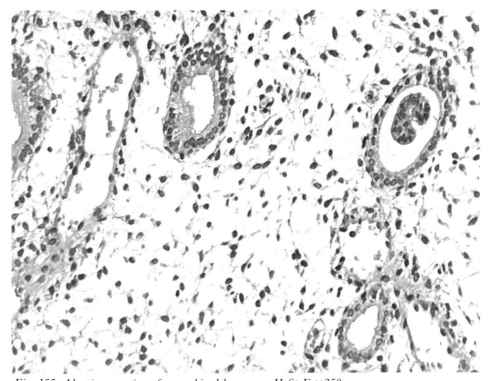

Fig. 155. Abortive secretion after combined hormones. H & E,×250.

Irregular atrophy (Fig. 156): Develops from abortive secretion when hormone therapy is continued for many months. Groups of glands become quite narrow and lined by atrophic epithelium until they disappear completely, whereas neighboring glands still remain in abortive secretion. The undifferentiated stroma is focally dense. The general height of the endometrium is decreased and the surface irregular.

Clinical correlation: Irregular atrophy is characteristic of longstanding hormone combination therapy. Rare endogenous causes (e.g. sudden cessation of estrogen secretion following irregular proliferation) must be excluded by the clinical history.

Break-through bleeding (Figs. 157 and 158): Results from focal dissolution of reticulin fibers due to the variations in hormone deficiency from area to area that depend on insufficient blood supply. Spiral arterioles fail to develop, yet small or dilated capillaries proliferate in areas of incomplete stromal differentiation (Ober 1966, 1977). The regional drop in hormone supply results in spotty, round hemorrhages characteristic of the artificial cycle.

Clinical correlation: The round circumscribed hemorrhages in an atrophic endometrium are characteristic of break-through bleeding under hormonal therapy. Anovulatory withdrawal bleeding from endogenous sources is more diffuse (cf. Figs. 78 and 79).

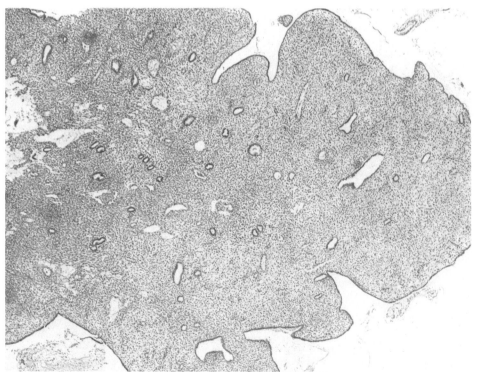

Fig. 156. *Irregular atrophy after combined hormones. H & E, ×25.*

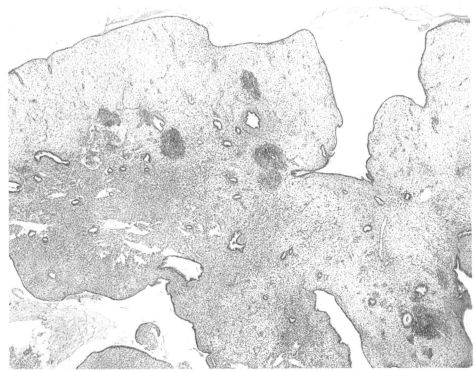

Fig. 157. Break-through bleeding. H & E,×25.

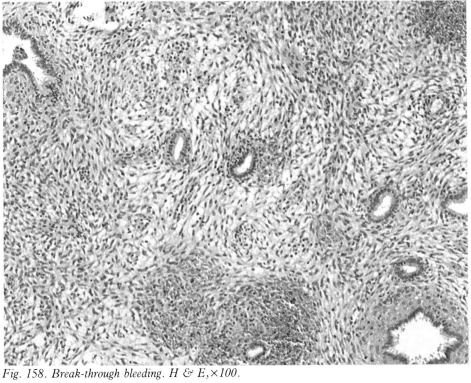

Fig. 158. Break-through bleeding. H & E,×100.

137

Irregular regeneration (Figs. 159 and 160): Occurs when oral contraceptives are discontinued. While some glands remain atrophic, others regenerate as in a normal cycle, but their shape and location vary. The stroma is densely cellular. The surface epithelium is focally low cuboidal, but in neighboring areas tall columnar (Fig. 160). The general height is quite irregular.

Clinical possibilities and differential diagnosis: a) Discontinuation of hormone therapy. b) Resumption of cyclic function following abortion or pregnancy.

Distinction is possible by evaluation of the clinical history.

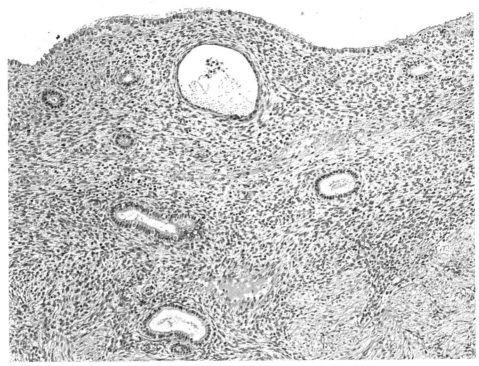

Fig. 159. Irregular regeneration following oral contraceptives. H & E, ×100.

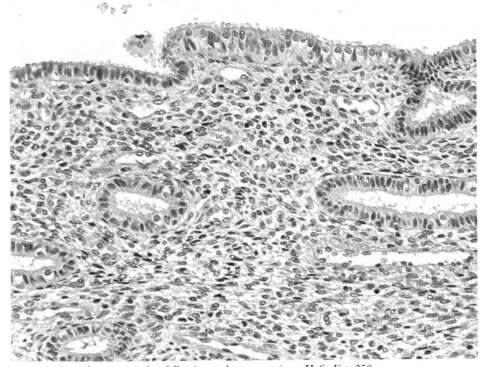

Fig. 160. Irregular regeneration following oral contraceptives. H & E, ×250.

Focal stromal hyperplasia (Figs. 161 and 162): Develops on rare occasions as an individual reaction to combined treatment with hormones. In these foci the stromal cells have hyperchromatic enlarged nuclei, and there is excessive formation of reticulin fibers. The number and the structure of the endometrial glands in these foci remain unaltered.

Morphologic differential diagnosis: These foci of iatrogenic stromal hyperplasia must be differentiated from the rare presarcomatous stromal hyperplasia (stromal nodule) which is a diffuse stromal proliferation with rarefaction of glands (see p. 190).

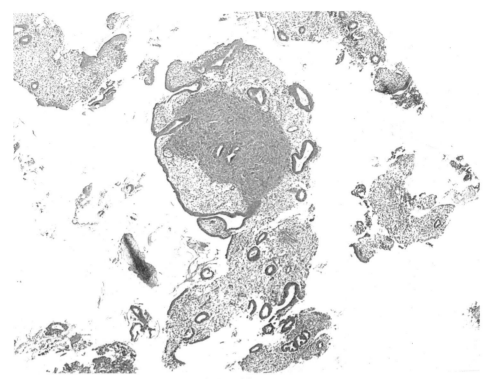

Fig. 161. Focal stromal hyperplasia. H & E,×25.

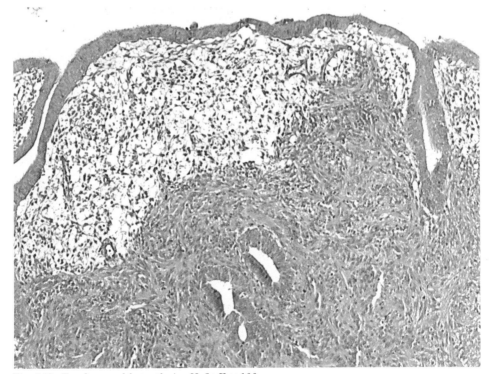

Fig. 162. Focal stromal hyperplasia. H & E,×100.

Pseudomelanosis (Figs. 163, 164 and 165): On gross examination the endometrial surface is sprinkled with tiny, grayish-black dots caused by the inspissation of blood in the slightly dilated glandular lumina. This change indicates that the endometrium has not been shed with menstruation. The glands have merely regenerated and been incorporated in the next cycle.

Clinical possibilities and differential diagnosis: Incomplete or absent menstrual shedding with inspissation of menstrual blood from the uterine cavity into the regenerating glands due to: a) Hormone therapy. b) Endogenous disturbance such as insufficient stromal differentiation with absence of endometrial granulocytes.

Distinction is possible by evaluation of the clinical history.

Focal adenomatous hyperplasia: May develop after prolonged treatment with agents that contain predominantly estrogen, particularly after sequential oral contraceptive agents, or after metabolic conversion of gestagens into compounds with estrogenic action (Charles 1964; Henzl et al. 1964). Structurally these foci are identical with the diffuse adenomatous hyperplasia (see Figs. 94-102).

The **early structural changes following sequential therapy** are identical to those of the deficient secretory phase with coordinated true delay of maturation (see p. 108).

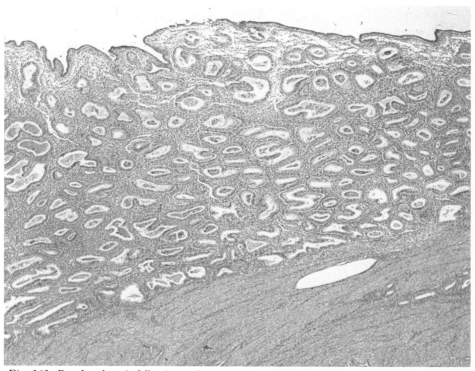

Fig. 163. Pseudomelanosis following oral contraceptives. H & E, ×25.

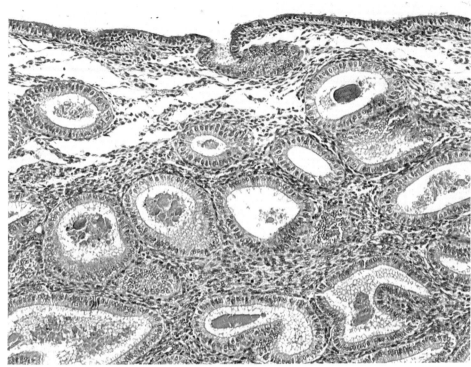

Fig. 164. Pseudomelanosis following oral contraceptives. H & E,×100.

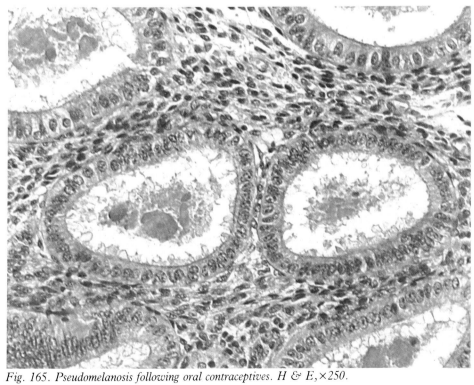

Fig. 165. Pseudomelanosis following oral contraceptives. H & E,×250.

After intrauterine contraceptive device

The histologic reaction of the endometrium to the device varies with the type used.

Mechanical decidualization

(Figs. 166 and 167). With the inert device, mechanical pressure or injury of endometrium results in early decidualization of the surrounding stroma, a change that can be observed shortly after ovulation (Wynn 1968). The endometrium directly beneath the device may show pressure atrophy with focal fibrosis and

occasional ulceration with perifocal inflammatory infiltrates (Fig. 166). The decidualization is limited to small foci and is surrounded by non-decidualized endometrium corresponding to the day of the cycle (Fig. 167).

Morphologic differential diagnosis: from early decidua of intra- or extrauterine pregnancy is necessary. Distinction is possible when previous insertion of IUD is known, or when one finds neighboring non-decidualized endometrium, proving the focal character of the decidual change. Arrested secretion can be excluded through the atrophy of its glands (see Figs. 148 and 149).

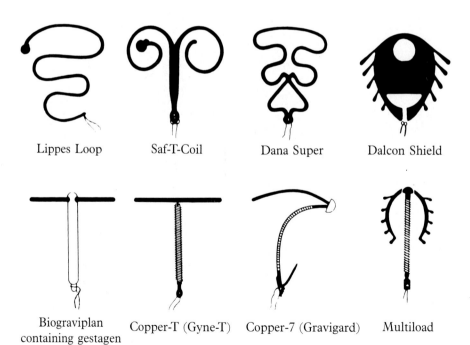

Lippes Loop   Saf-T-Coil   Dana Super   Dalcon Shield

Biograviplan containing gestagen   Copper-T (Gyne-T)   Copper-7 (Gravigard)   Multiload

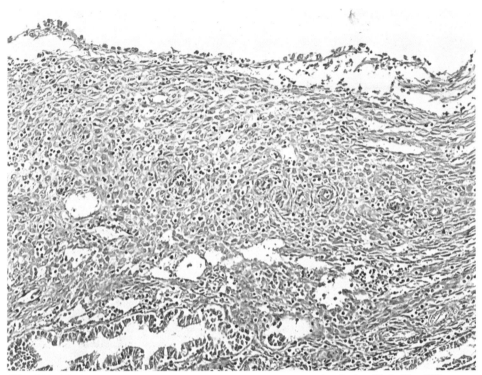

Fig. 166. Mechanical decidualization after intrauterine contraceptive device. H & E,×100.

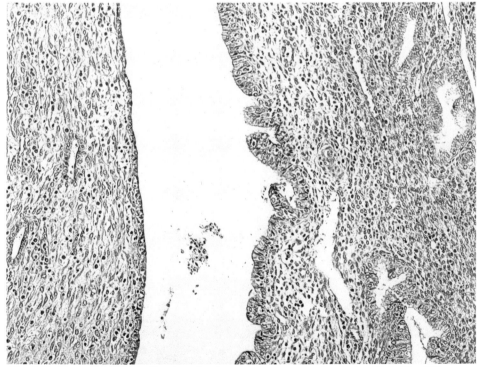

Fig. 167. Mechanical decidualization after intrauterine contraceptive device. H & E,×100.

Perifocal arrested secretion

(Figs. 168 and 169). The progesterone-medicated devices release small amounts of the hormone from the depot into the uterine cavity. The gestagen penetrates into the endometrium and acts locally in a paracrine manner. The diffusion only reaches the superficial layers and ends with a discrete horizontal line which can be seen on histologic examination (Fig. 168): The upper compact layer shows very sparse, narrow, atrophic glands surrounded by decidualized stroma (Fig. 169). Sinusoidal spaces are cystically dilated. Surface indentations indicate pressure by the device (Fig. 168). This perifocal arrested secretion presents the same morphologic and histochemical changes as diffuse arrested secretion (Johannisson et al. 1977; cf. Figs. 148 and 149), but without systemic effects (Wan et al. 1977). Beneath the decidualized layer one finds unaffected endometrial glands and stroma corresponding to the day of the cycle.

Morphologic differential diagnosis: Possible from: a) Arrested secretion induced by administration of gestagens orally or parenterally, which involves the entire endometrium. b) Mechanical decidualization brought about by pressure or trauma of a mechanical device: this condition resembles a normal decidua with secretory glands but is focally limited.

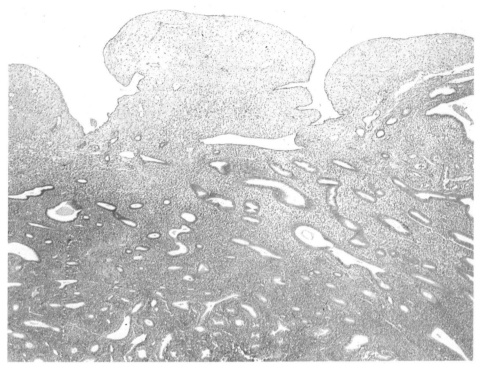

Fig. 168. Perifocal arrested secretion following gestagen-laden device. H & E,×25.

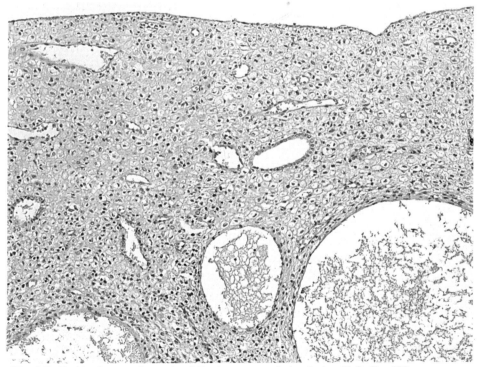

Fig. 169. Perifocal arrested secretion following gestagen-laden device. H & E,×100.

Surface reaction following copper devices

(Figs. 170, 171 and 172). The devices entwined with a copper wire cause regular pressure indentations in the endometrium, the size of the wire used resulting in a corrugated endometrial surface. There is slight pressure atrophy directly underneath the wire, but the surface epithelium generally remains intact (Fig. 172). Except for a dysfunctional endometrium, no inflammatory changes are found. The endometrium of uteri bearing this type of device remains morphologically unchanged presenting a normal secretory (Fig. 170) or proliferative phase (Fig. 171). The contraceptive action apparently comes about by biochemical changes (Rosado et al. 1976; Wilson 1977).

Clinical correlation: The corrugated endometrial surface is seen only after insertion of a copper device.

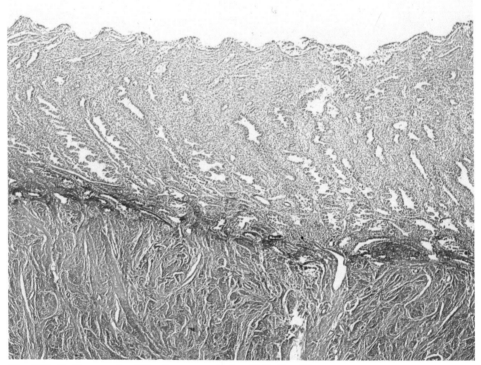

Fig. 170. Surface reaction following copper device. H & E,×25.

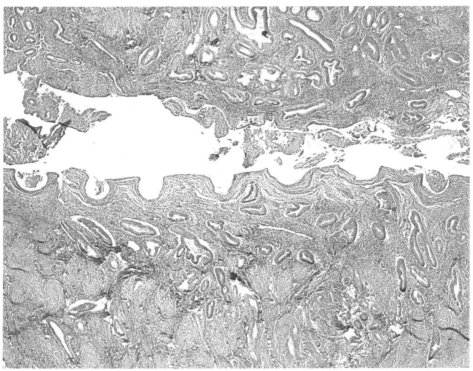

Fig. 171. Surface reaction following copper device. H & E, ×25.

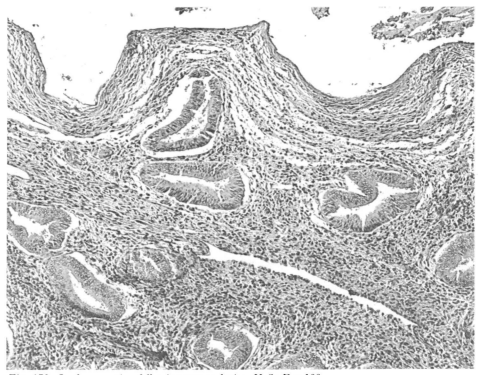

Fig. 172. Surface reaction following copper device. H & E, ×100.

Leukocytes in glandular lumina

(Figs. 173 and 174). Leukocytes in glandular lumina indicate that a copper device has been inserted. They are pushed into the glandular mouth (Fig. 173) of normally secreting glands. There is no inflammatory reaction of the glandular epithelium or stroma. Note the intact surface epithelium. These leukocytes are thus of no clinical importance.

Morphologic differential diagnosis is necessary from endometritis, which shows glandular and stromal infiltration by inflammatory cells.

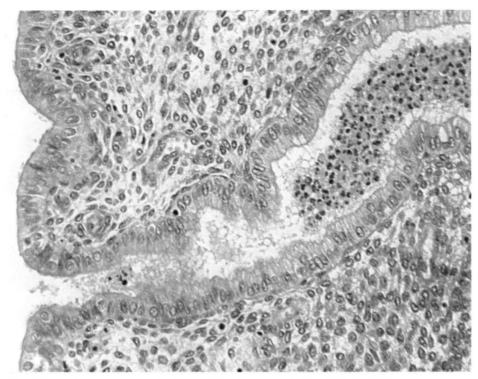

Fig. 173. Leukocytes in glandular lumina following copper device. H & E,×250.

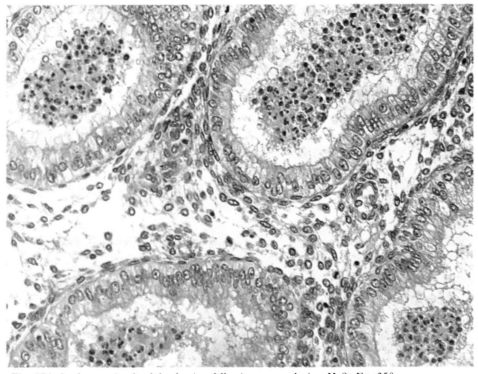

Fig. 174. Leukocytes in glandular lumina following copper device. H & E,×250.

After intrauterine instillation

When a contrast medium (for hysterosalpingo-graphy) or a liquid adhesive (for permanent sterilization) is instilled into the uterine cavity, various histologic changes may develop.

Histiocytic storage reaction

(Figs. 175, 176 and 177). In hyperplastic endometria that do not shed cyclically, histiocytes may incorporate the material that has been pressed into the superficial stroma. Patches of necrotic material can be seen in the stroma between cystically dilated glands and surrounded by small histiocytes, and partly incorporated by large macrophages laden with a foamy substance which displaces their nuclei (Fig. 177).

Morphologic differential diagnosis is necessary from: a) Foci of epithelial or stromal metaplasia. b) Neoplastic cells. Distinction is possible by careful examination of these foci and by applying special stains to identify cells and accumulations.

Clinical correlation and differential diagnosis: Since this storage is usually an incidental finding it may be difficult to explain clinically.

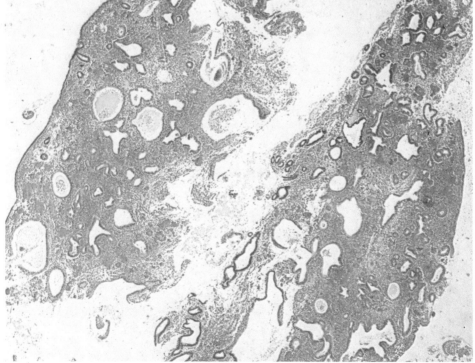

Fig. 175. Histiocytic storage reaction. H & E, ×25.

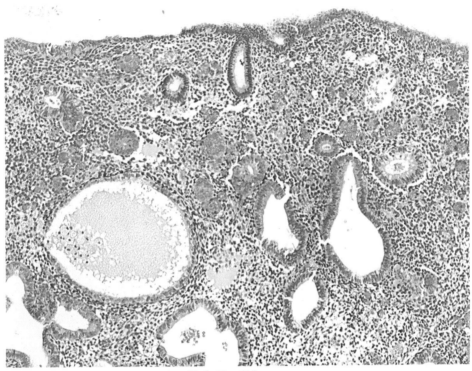

Fig. 176. Histiocytic storage reaction. H & E, ×100.

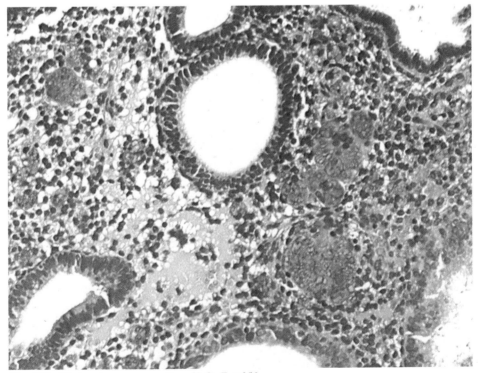

Fig. 177. Histiocytic storage reaction. H & E, ×250.

CHAPTER 6

Endometritis

Acute endometritis

(Figs. 178, 179 and 180). Although the causative agents are numerous, the inflammatory reactions to them are generally the same. Stroma and glands are diffusely or focally infiltrated with polymorphonuclear leukocytes intermixed with lymphocytes and occasional plasma cells. The surface and glandular epithelia are more or less destroyed by the heavy infiltrates, and the reticulin fibers of the stroma disintegrate. There are areas of hemorrhage or edema in the stroma. The cyclic function of the endometrium is often preserved. The infected portions of the endometrium may be shed with the next menstruation unless the basal layer is also involved.

Morhologic differential diagnosis: Distinction of the inflammatory infiltrates from endometrial granulocytes is necessary: the endometrial granulocytes, which closely resemble polymorphonuclear leukocytes in shape, do not penetrate or destroy the glandular epithelium. Furthermore, areas of hemorrhagic necrosis, occurring in endometria with protracted shedding in functional disorders, should not be misinterpreted as signs of endometritis.

Clinical possibilities and differential diag-

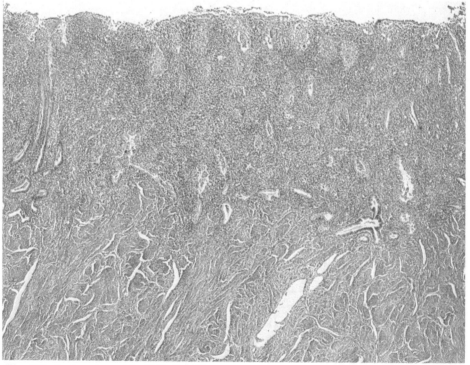

Fig. 178. Acute endometritis. H & E, ×25.

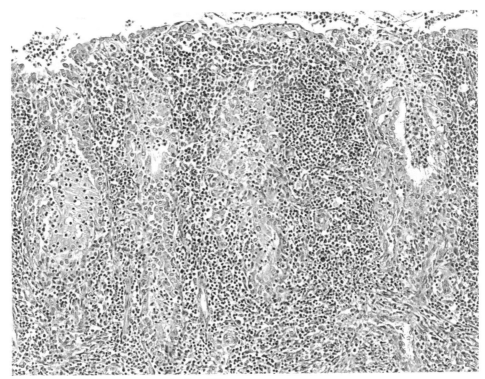

Fig. 179. Acute endometritis. H & E, ×100.

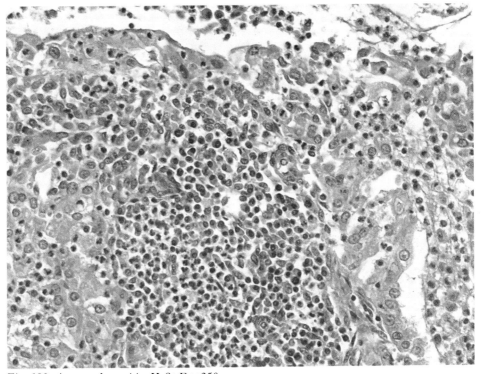

Fig. 180. Acute endometritis. H & E, ×250.

nosis: Acute endometritis occurs as an ascending infection when the cervical barrier is damaged: a) Most frequently in abortion. b) Following menses, delivery, curettage or insertion of an IUD. Endometritis post abortum can be recognized from the characteristic changes óf the endometrial glands (irregular shedding: cf. Figs. 125-128), remnants of decidua and possibly placental villi or trophoblasts.

Chronic non-specific endometritis

(Figs. 181, 182 and 183). Endometritis can only become chronic when the endometrium does not shed with menstruation. Hence, the endometrial glands are hyperplastic, irregularly or insufficiently proliferated, resting or atrophic, and the stromal cells are spindle-shaped. The inflammatory infiltrates mainly consist of lymphocytes and plasma cells, which are scattered diffusely throughout the stroma or aggregated focally. They also infiltrate and destroy the glandular and surface epithelium. There is, however, no destruction of reticulin fibers, and the endometrial architecture is preserved.

Morphologic differential diagnosis: Lymphocytic infiltrates without glandular involvement in the absence of plasma cells are not diagnostic for chronic endometritis, but may occur physiologically. On the other hand, chronic non-specific endometritis must be differentiated from tuberculous endometritis, which may have lost most of its characteristic granulomatous reaction with Langhans giant cells. Careful search for epithelioid tubercles is necessary to exclude such a possibility.

Clinical correlation and differential diagnosis: The causative agents are the same as in acute infection. In senile patients chronic endometritis easily develops in low resistant atrophic endometrium and may be associated with necrotic polyps or carcinoma.

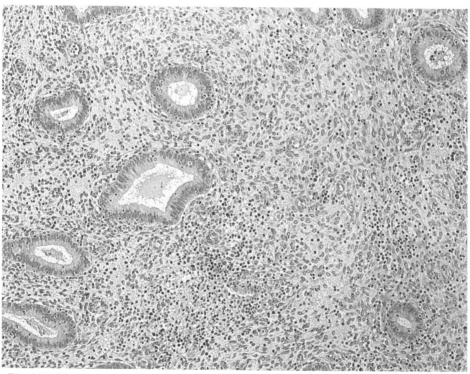

Fig. 181. Chronic non-specific endometritis. H & E, ×100.

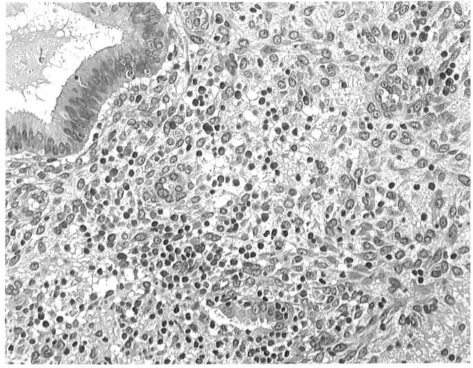

Fig. 182. Chronic non-specific endometritis. H & E, ×250.

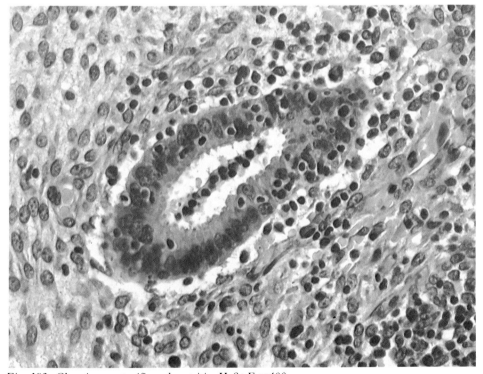

Fig. 183. Chronic non-specific endometritis. H & E, ×400.

Tuberculous endometritis

(Figs. 184 and 185). The extent of the involvement of the endometrium may vary greatly. In servere infection typical granulomas with Langhans giant cells and epithelioid cells surrounded by lymphocytes are crowded together to varying extents, filling large portions of the stroma (Fig. 184) and protruding into glandular lumina. There may be caseous necrosis and ulceration of the endometrial surface. The glandular epithelium often responds by atypical proliferation, stratification, metaplasia or new gland formation. The endometrial function is disturbed, the peritubercular fibrosis inhibits endometrial shedding.

Morphologic differential diagnosis is necessary from similar specific granulomas such as sarcoidosis and mycotic infections, and from foreign body granuloma. Sarcoidosis contains no acid-fast bacteria and shows no caseation. In mycotic granulomas fungal organisms can often be found by special stains. Foreign body granulomas often can be recognized by their birefringent material under polarizing illumination.

Clinical correlation: Endometrial involvement occurs from tuberculous bacteria descending from a tuberculous salpingitis.

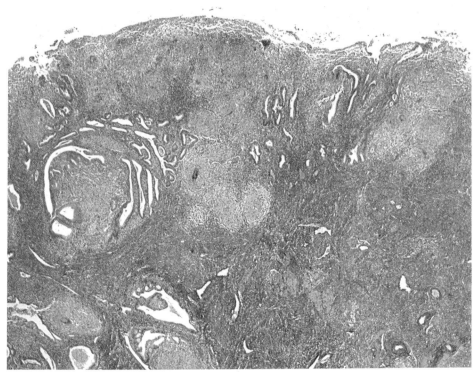

Fig. 184. Tuberculous endometritis. H & E, ×25.

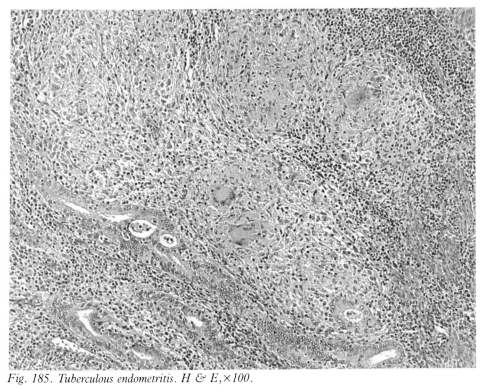

Fig. 185. Tuberculous endometritis. H & E, ×100.

159

Sarcoidosis

(Figs. 186 and 187). Granulomas consisting of epithelioid cells and usually multinucleated giant cells closely resembling tuberculous granulomas occupy areas of the endometrial stroma. In contrast to tuberculosis, there is no caseation, and glandular involvement or reactive hyperproliferation is very rare. The endometria involved are often diffusely hyperplastic (Fig. 186) since they do not shed with menstruation.

Morphologic differential diagnosis: Tuberculous or related granulomas, see p. 158.

Clinical correlation and differential diagnosis: Endometrial involvement in a systemic sarcoidosis is rare, but differentiation from tuberculosis is of clinical importance.

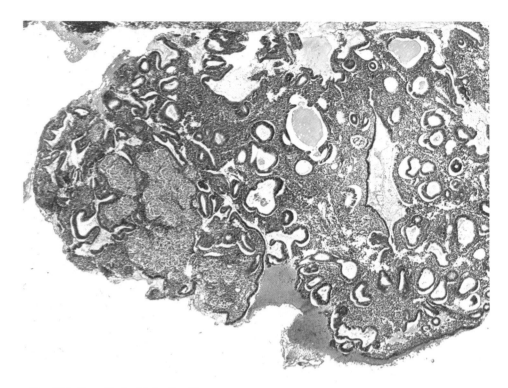

Fig. 186. Sarcoidosis. H & E,×25.

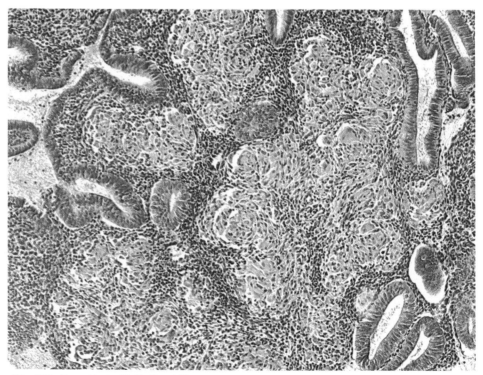

Fig. 187. Sarcoidosis. H & E,×100.

Actinomycosis

(Figs. 188 and 189). Characteristic radiating particles of various sizes can be found between endometrial fragments disintegrated by inflammatory infiltrates.

Clinical correlation: Actinomyces infection of the endometrium is a rare complication after insertion of an intrauterine contraceptive device (Lomax et el. 1976).

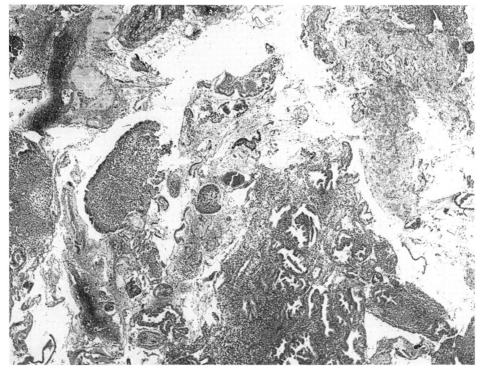

Fig. 188. Actinomycosis. H & E, ×25.

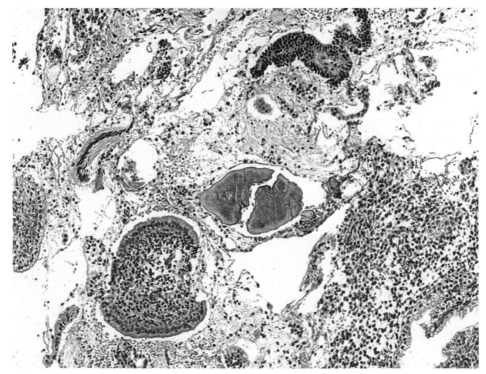

Fig. 189. Actinomycosis. H & E, ×100.

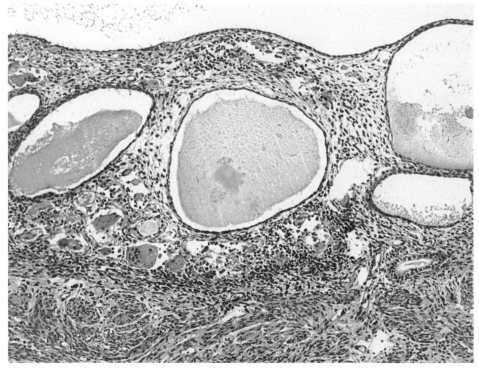

Fig. 190. Foreign body granuloma. H & E,×100.

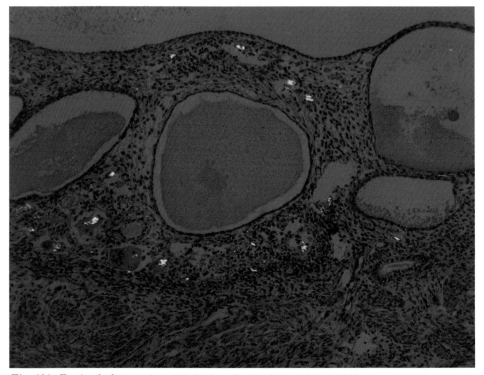

Fig. 191. Foreign body granuloma. H & E under bipolarized light, ×100.

Foreign body granuloma

(Figs. 190, 191 and 192). Resting or cystic atrophic endometria that do not shed may harbor foreign body granulomas, preferably in the basal layer (Fig. 190), consisting of multinucleated foreign body giant cells surrounded by chronic inflammatory infiltrates. The giant cells may contain variously shaped birefringent crystals (Fig. 191) which they have phagocytized (Fig. 192).

Morphologic differential diagnosis: Similar granulomas, see p. 158. The presence of birefringent inclusions under polarized light is diagnostic.

Clinical correlation: Talcum granulomas may develop after intrauterine procedures. Foreign body granulomas caused by other materials are rare in the endometrium.

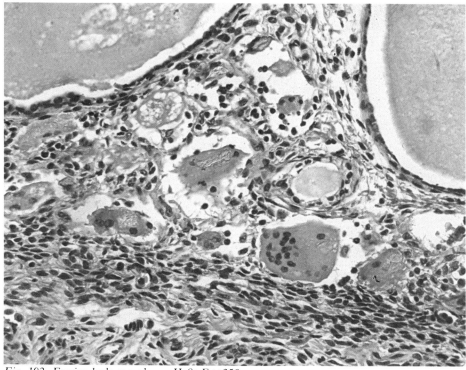

Fig. 192. Foreign body granuloma. H & E, ×250.

CHAPTER 7

Neoplasms

Carcinomas

According to histogenetic principles the carcinomas of the endometrium can be subdivided into those of endometrial origin (adenocarcinoma and adenocarcinoma with squamous metaplasia (mature and immature)) and those from pluripotential Müllerian epithelium (carcinomas of endocervical type (mucinous and mucoepidermoid carcinoma), clear cell carcinoma, papillary carcinoma and squamous cell carcinoma).

In the characterization of endometrial carcinomas there are three possibilities: Histologic typing, grading of differentiation, and staging, (Poulsen et al. 1975). These are especially important in the endometrial type of adenocarcinoma which can be subdivided into the common type, the secretory type, and the estrogen type. Grading (Grades I-III) is only of prognostic value in the endometrial type of adenocarcinoma and in papillary carcinoma. Staging, estimation of extent of tumor growth, is of importance for all categories of carcinoma.

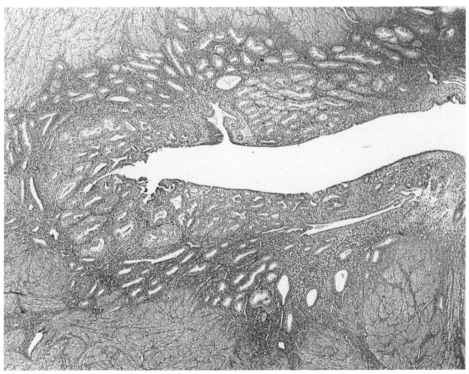

Fig. 193. Early adenocarcinoma. H & E, ×25.

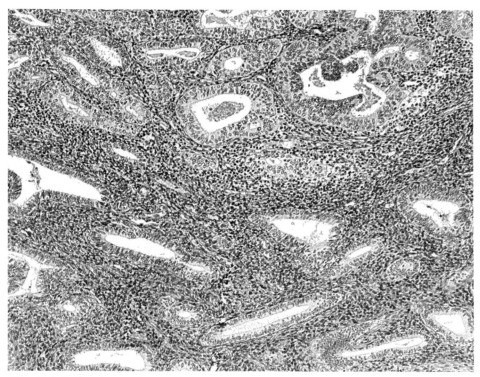

Fig. 194. Early adenocarcinoma. H & E, ×100.

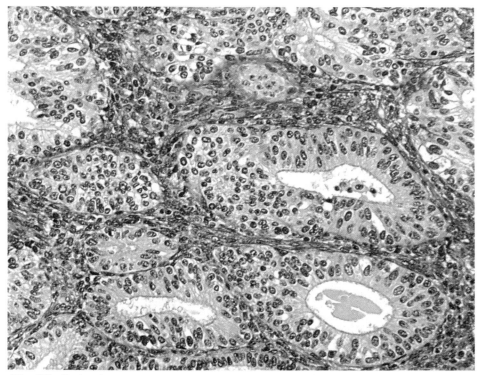

Fig. 195. Early adenocarcinoma. H & E, ×250.

Adenocarcinoma

Early adenocarcinoma (Figs. 193, 194 and 195): Early carcinomatous changes may develop focally or multicentrically within an adenomatous hyperplasia. They are always limited to the endometrium (Fig. 193). Within these foci, groups of glands are lined by multilayered, atypical epithelial cells which have depolarized, enlarged nuclei containing prominent nucleoli. They are frequently in mitosis. Their cytoplasm is pale or vacuolated (Fig. 195). The stroma is rarefied and focally scant, particularly in regions with microalveolar change. The early carcinomatous foci have compressed borders and may be surrounded by lymphocytic infiltrates indicating stromal invasion (Fig. 194). Most of these early carcinomas are glandular Grade I, but occasionally Grade II or even Grade III may be seen.

Morphologic differential diagnosis: Early adenocarcinoma has to be differentiated from Grade III adenomatous hyperplasia (cf. Figs. 100-102). The most important criterion for the beginning of carcinomatous growth is stromal invasion (Kurman and Norris 1982). According to these authors the main criteria for invasion are: a desmoplastic stromal reaction around irregularly infiltrating glands, a confluent glandular pattern with microalveolar proliferation and loss of stroma, an extensive papillary pattern or large areas of squamous metaplasia. One of these criteria, if it occupies one half of a low power field, would be sufficient for a diagnosis of stromal invasion.

Well differentiated adenocarcinoma (FIGO Grade I) (Figs. 196 and 197): The well differentiated tubular glands appear slender, contain little or no mucus (Fig. 196), and are lined by pseudostratified or stratified epithelial cells with elongated large nuclei, prominent nucleoli and frequent mitoses (Fig. 197). Their cytoplasm is sparse. A few papillary structures may be seen (see p. 188). The stroma between the glands is reduced to scanty fibers of collagen and thin capillaries.

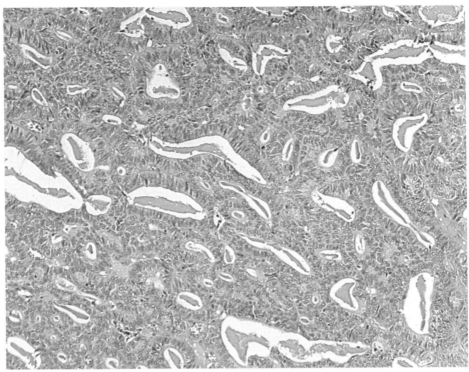

Fig. 196. Well differentiated adenocarcinoma (Grade I), H & E, ×100.

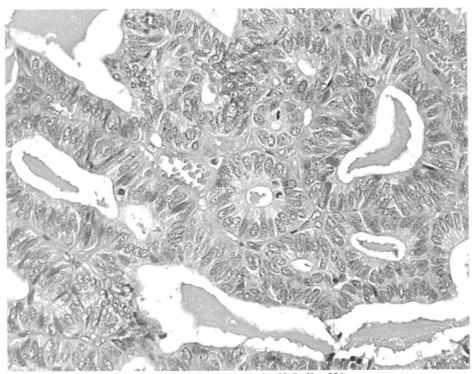

Fig. 197. Well differentiated adenocarcinoma (Grade I), H & E, ×250.

Partly undifferentiated adenocarcinoma (FIGO Grade II) (Figs. 198, 199 and 200): Whereas some areas of these carcinomas are well differentiated as in Fig. 196 and 197, neighboring areas consist of solid sheets of cells. The nuclei in these areas are depolarized or form pseudorosettes, indicating early stages of microglandular formation (Fig. 200). There may be a sharp line between well differentiated and undifferentiated carcinomatous areas (Figs. 198 and 199). On the other hand, the FIGO category Grade II also includes moderately differentiated adenocarcinomas without focal variation in the degree of differentiation.

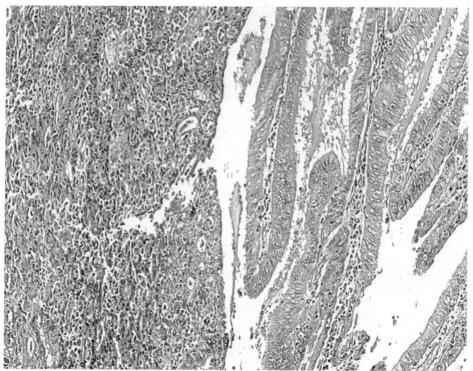

Fig. 198. Partly undifferentiated adenocarcinoma (Grade II), H & E,×100.

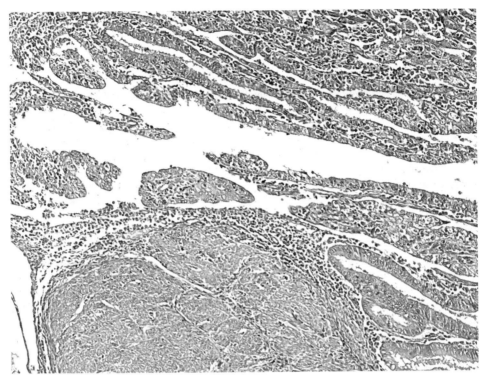

Fig. 199. Partly undifferentiated adenocarcinoma (Grade II), H & E,×100.

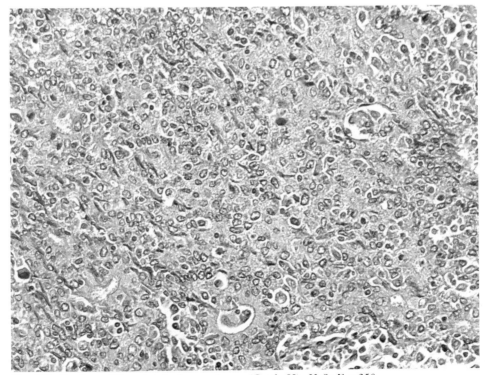

Fig. 200. Partly undifferentiated adenocarcinoma (Grade II), H & E,×250.

171

Undifferentiated solid adenocarcinoma (FIGO Grade III) (Figs. 201 and 202): These carcinomas consist only of solid areas of undifferentiated carcinomatous cells, which are disorderly arranged in large portions. In some foci pseudorosettes may be distinguished, indicating the adenomatous nature of the tumor. This criterion can be used to differentiate the solid adenocarcinoma from an undifferentiated squamous cell carcinoma.

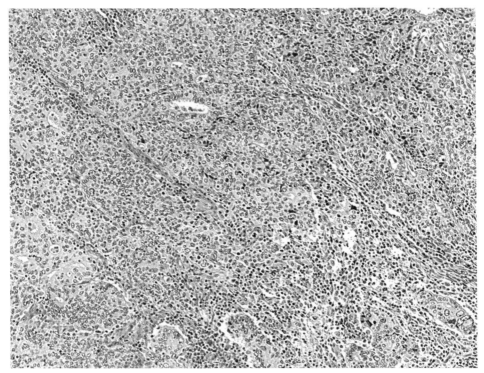

Fig. 201. Undifferentiated solid adenocarcinoma (Grade III), H & E, ×100.

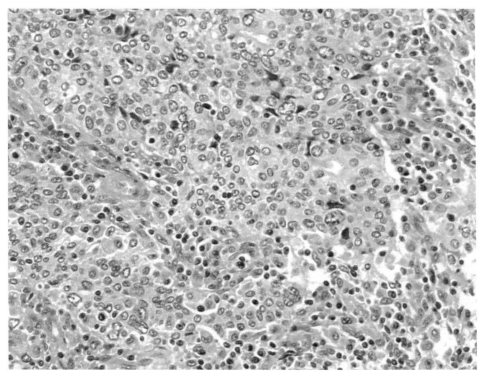

Fig. 202. Undifferentiated solid adenocarcinoma (Grade III), H & E, ×250.

Secretory adenocarcinoma (Figs. 203, 204 and 205): This is a well differentiated adenocarcinoma with convoluted glands containing cells with irregular, depolarized nuclei often in a single row in abundant secreting cytoplasm. Except for this pronounced secretory change, there is no remarkable difference between this type of carcinoma and the well differentiated type of adenocarcinoma (cf. Figs. 196 and 197).

Clinical correlation: The secretory adenocarcinoma is rare. Some patients with these tumors have been treated with high doses of gestagen, which explains the secretory activity of the glandular epithelium (cf. Figs. 151 and 152). In the remaining patients, the source for this progestational effect may be difficult to clarify, since most of them are in the late post-menopause (Christopherson et al. 1982 a, b).

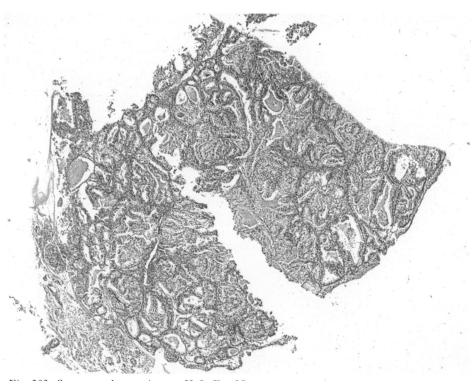

Fig. 203. Secretory adenocarcinoma. H & E, ×25.

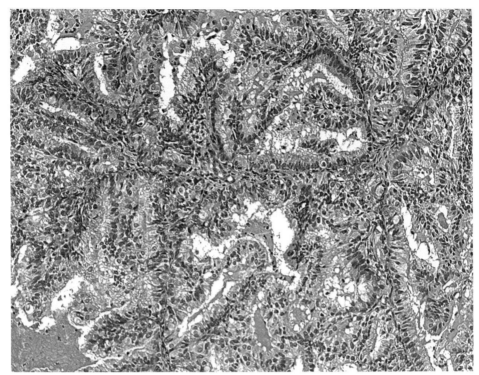

Fig. 204. Secretory adenocarcinoma. H & E, ×100.

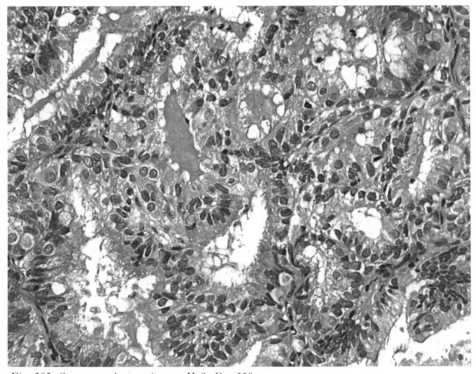

Fig. 205. Secretory adenocarcinoma. H & E, ×250.

175

Estrogen type of adenocarcinoma (Figs. 206, 207 and 208): The adenocarcinomas developing under the influence of exogenous estrogen often present a characteristic pattern that inspired the name "estrogen-carcinomas" (Gusberg and Hall 1961). A high percentage of these carcinomas contain nodules or accumulations of squamous epithelium (Robboy and Bradley 1979). Most of the carcinomatous glands are well differentiated but may vary in their structure from area to area (Fig. 207), some being cystically dilated with branching intraluminal epithelial papillae (Fig. 206). Accumulations of endometrial foam cells between the carcinomatous glands are frequently encountered.

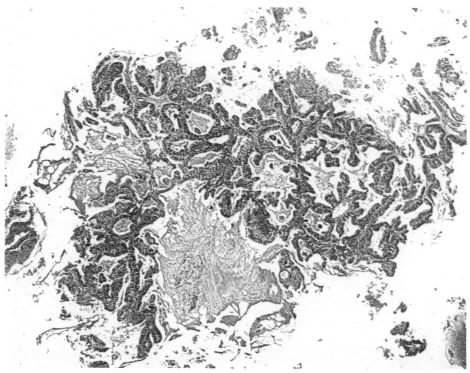

Fig. 206. Estrogen type of adenocarcinoma. H & E, ×25.

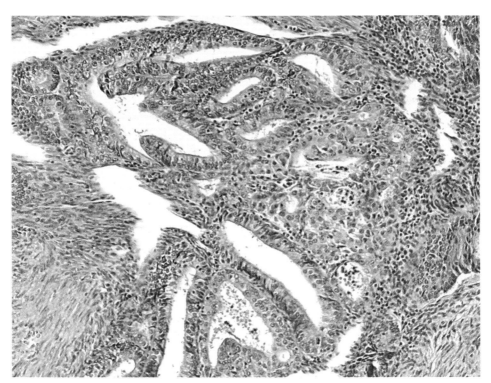

Fig. 207. Estrogen type of adenocarcinoma. H & E, ×100.

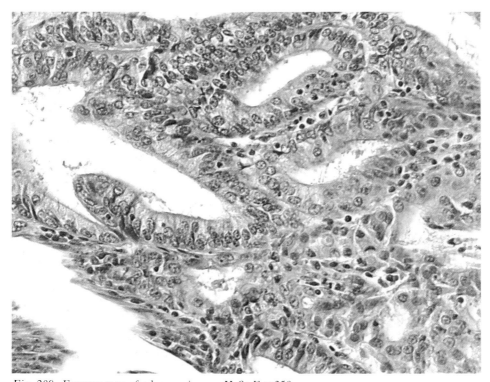

Fig. 208. Estrogen type of adenocarcinoma. H & E, ×250.

Adenocarcinoma with squamous metaplasia

This term includes adenocarcinomas with mature as well as with immature squamous metaplasia.

Adenoacanthoma

(Figs. 209, 210 and 211). This is nearly always a well differentiated adenocarcinoma of the endometrial type which contains nodules as well as islets of mature squamous epithelium. Some nodules contain parakeratotic horn pearls; others reveal intracellular bridges (Fig. 211). The carcinomatous glands may also grow in a papillary fashion, but, in contrast to the papillary carcinoma, they maintain their stratified glandular structure.

Morphologic differential diagnosis: Adenoacanthoma must be differentiated from adenosquamos carcinoma (see p. 180) because of its far more favorable prognosis (Connelly et al. 1982). The 5-year survival rate of patients with adenoacanthoma is 87%, that of patients with adenosquamous carcinoma is only 47%.

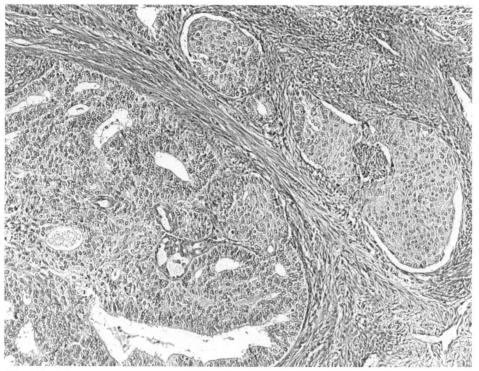

Fig. 209. Adenoacanthoma (adenocarcinoma with mature squamous metaplasia). H & E, ×100.

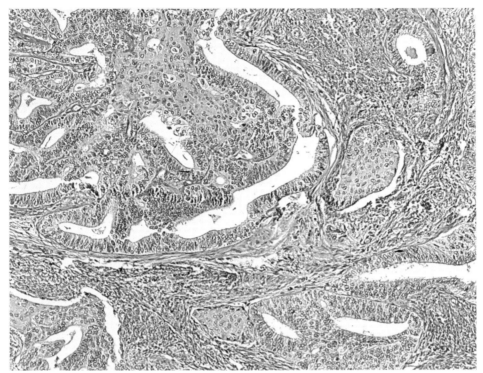

Fig. 210. Adenoacanthoma (adenocarcinoma with mature squamous metaplasia). H & E, ×100.

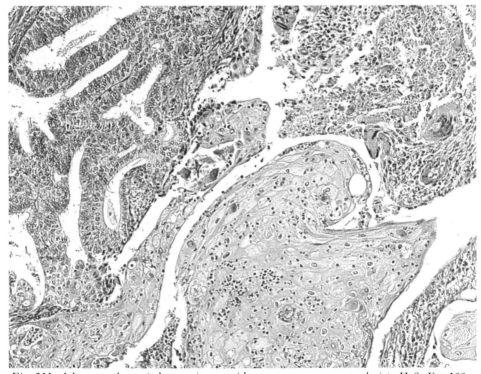

Fig. 211. Adenoacanthoma (adenocarcinoma with mature squamous metaplasia). H & E, ×100.

Adenosquamous Carcinoma

(Figs. 212 and 213). In this carcinoma there is an intimate mixture of glandular and solid epithelial structures. Some glands are more or less well differentiated, others microalveolar. The solid areas consist of immature squamous elements with atypical nuclei, frequent mitoses, and fairly abundant eosinophilic cytoplasm.

Morphologic differential diagnosis: Adenoacanthoma: the most important clue for distinction is the irregularity in distribution and the immaturity of the squamous component; only carcinomas with nodules of mature squamous metaplasia should be called adenoacanthoma. The nuclei of the squamous cells in adenoacanthoma reveal diploid DNA measurements, whereas those in adenosquamous carcinoma have aneuploid values. In addition, the glandular component in adenosquamous carcinoma is usually much less well differentiated than in adenoacanthoma and usually does not contain mucin.

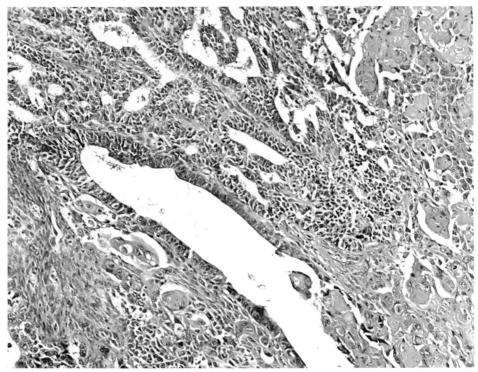

Fig. 212. Adenosquamous carcinoma. H & E, ×100.

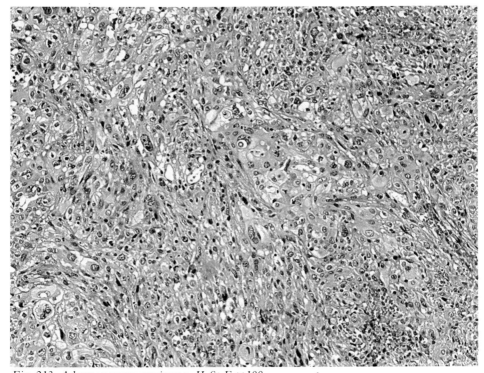

Fig. 213. Adenosquamous carcinoma. H & E, ×100.

Carcinoma of Endocervical Type

These carcinomas most likely develop from foci of endocervical metaplasia (see p. 56).

Mucinous Carcinoma

The mucinous adenocarcinoma closely resembles a mature adenocarcinoma of the endocervical mucosa. Its histological structure corresponds to the well differentiated adenomatous portions of the mucoepidermoid adenocarcinoma (see below). Its morphological distinction from a primary endocervical adenocarcinoma may be impossible from curettings.

Mucoepidermoid Carcinoma

The mucoepidermoid adenocarcinoma (Figs. 214 and 215) shows mucus formation in some of the glands which may be cystically dilated. Occasionally intracellular mucin is also found.

The squamous areas may contain horn pearls or develop monocellular keratinization, and in addition show a general cellular pleomorphism.

Morphologic differential diagnosis: Mucoepidermoid adenocarcinoma of the endocervix: this distinction may prove to be extremely difficult, if not impossible, from curretings consisting of only carcinomatous tissue. A fractionated abrasio may help, but it is not fully reliable. An important factor may be the age of the patient: mucoepidermoid adenocarcinoma of the endometrium occurs predominantly in old age, often beyond the age of 70, whereas mucoepidermoid adenocarcinoma of the endocervix is found in women with an average age of 39 years (Dallenbach-Hellweg 1982). The distinction can be made with much more accuracy when the hysterectomy specimen is available for examination.

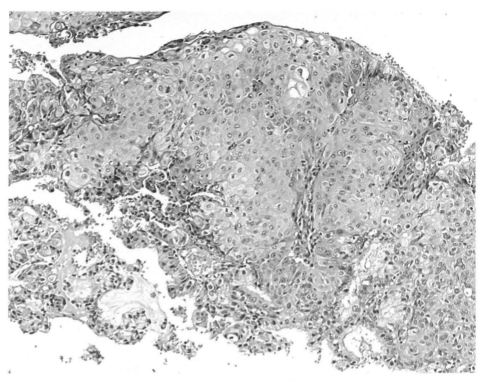

Fig. 214. Mucoepidermoid adenocarcinoma. H & E,×100.

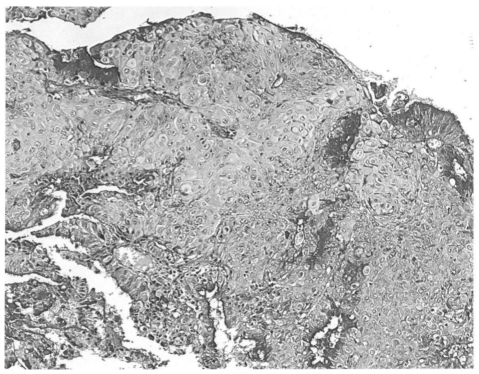

Fig. 215. Mucoepidermoid adenocarcinoma. PAS-reaction, ×100.

Clear cell carcinoma

(Figs. 216-219). This type of endometrial carcinoma looks very much like the clear cell carcinomas of the ovary, cervix and vagina (Silverberg and DeGiorgi 1973; Rorat et al. 1974; Roth 1974; Kurman and Scully 1976; Horie et al. 1977). Clear cell carcinoma is suggested to rise from the endocervical type epithelium but this has not been proven beyond doubt. The clear cells may be arranged in either *solid sheets* (Figs. 216 and 217), or may form cystic and tubular *glands* or *papillae* (Figs. 218 and 219). The large nuclei have irregular shapes and chromatin densities. Mitoses are frequent, but vary from region to region. The clear cytoplasm may contain glycogen or round PAS-positive and diastase-resistant hyaline inclusions (Christopherson et al. 1982). The cells forming papillae are often hobnail in shape (Fig. 219).

Morphologic differential diagnosis: From clear cell carcinoma of the endocervix may be impossible. For distinction the same criteria as for mucoepidermoid adenocarcinoma are valid (see above).

Clinical correlation: Histologic grading is of no importance, since all grades have an equally poor clinical prognosis with a 5-year survival rate of only 35%.

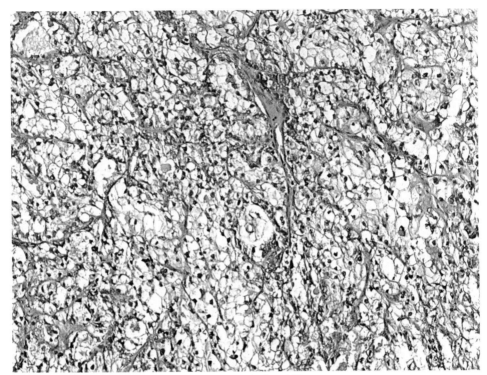

Fig. 216. Clear cell carcinoma, solid pattern. H & E, ×100.

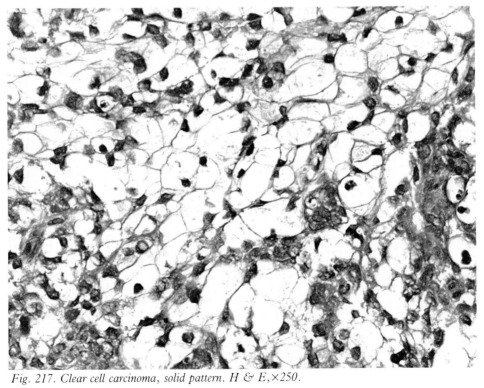

Fig. 217. Clear cell carcinoma, solid pattern. H & E, ×250.

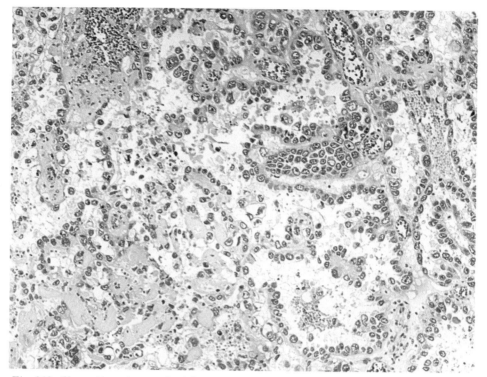

Fig. 218. Clear cell carcinoma, glandular papillary pattern. H & E, ×100.

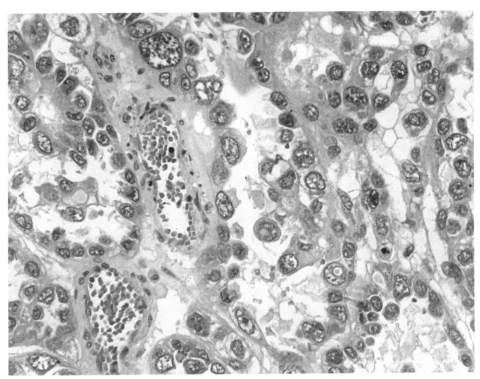

Fig. 219. Clear cell carcinoma, glandular papillary pattern. H & E, ×250.

Papillary carcinoma

(Figs. 220, 221 and 222). This carcinoma consists almost exclusively of long branching papillae with slim central stalks of connective tissue. The lining epithelial cells are columnar and contain elongated or rounded nuclei with varying densities of chromatin in an eosinophilic cytoplasm (Fig. 222). These tumors generally grow expansively into the uterine cavity (Fig. 220), often develop in polyps, and infiltrate the myometrium at a late stage. Nonetheless, their prognosis is less favorable than for the endometrial type of adenocarcinoma with a 5-year survival rate of 51% (Christopherson et al. 1982).

Morphologic differential diagnosis is of clinical importance from: a) Papillary formations in the well differentiated endometrial type of adenocarcinoma, in which the papillae are coarser and the cells are regularly arranged; b) Papillary type of clear cell carcinoma which presents hobnail formation of nuclei and intracytoplasmic hyaline inclusions.

Squamous cell carcinoma

This very rare type of carcinoma is seldom primary, and nearly always secondary (cf. Fig. 257).

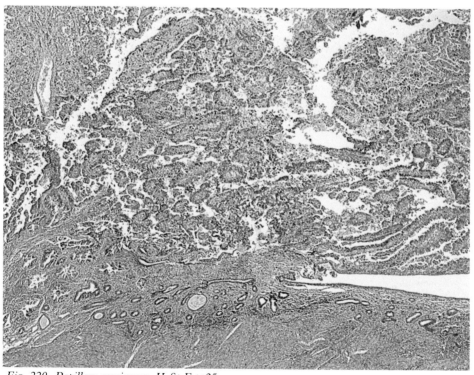

Fig. 220. Papillary carcinoma. H & E, ×25.

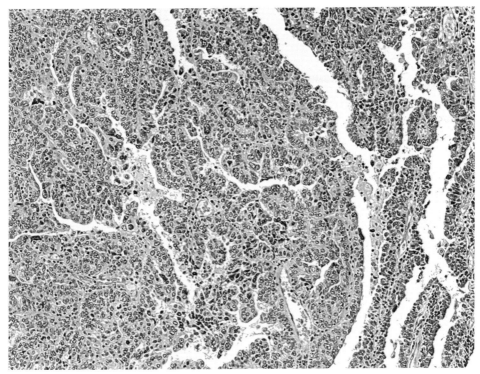

Fig. 221. Papillary carcinoma. H & E, ×100.

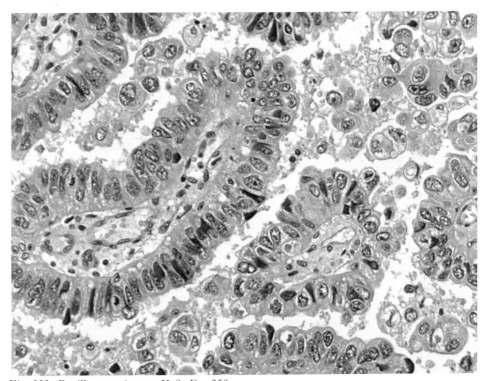

Fig. 222. Papillary carcinoma. H & E, ×250.

189

Stromal tumors

Stromal nodule (Focal stromal hyperplasia)

(Fig. 223). This rare, well circumscribed tumor may be located in the endometrium or myometrium; about 5% are multiple (Tavassoli and Norris 1981). Histologically, they are composed of uniform cells closely resembling normal endometrial stromal cells. Mitotic activity is low. Individual cells are enveloped by a dense reticulin network and occasionally by ribbons of hyalinized collagen. The cells are diffusely arranged (Fig. 223) or form small cords which may have a gland-like appearance. There are no glands, however. The nodules have rather sharp borders compressing the adjacent endometrium or myometrium. They are claimed to be benign, but may occasionally be presarcomatous (see p. 140).

Morphologic differential diagnosis is necessary from stromal sarcoma and endolymphatic stromal myosis. Both of these lesions have a much higher mitotic activity, infiltrate the endometrium and myometrium and grow in lymphatics and blood vessels.

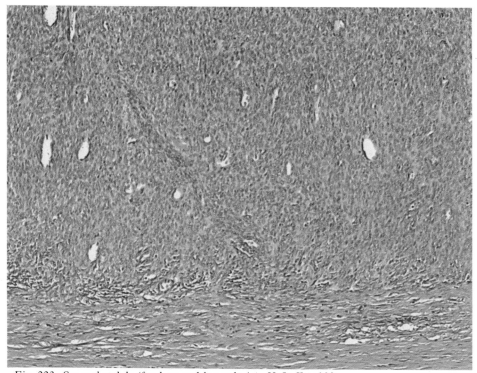

Fig. 223. Stromal nodule (focal stromal hyperplasia). H & E, ×100.

Stromal sarcoma (high grade)

The homologous type (Fig. 224-228): Consists of densely arranged *uniform* cells resembling the stromal cells of the early proliferative phase (Komorowski et al. 1970; Akhtar et al. 1975). Their round or oval nuclei are densely arranged. Usually more than 10 mitoses per 10 HPF can be counted (Norris and Taylor 1966; Fig. 226). The cytoplasm is sparse and appears immature (Böcker and Stegner 1975). The reticulin network varies and may be poorly developed in some areas. Endometrial glands are very sparse and absent in large regions. Some homologous stromal sarcomas show a *plexiform* pattern in which the cellular arrangement is not uniform, but condensed in branching cords which may resemble gonadal stroma in some areas (Clement and Scully 1976; Tang et al. 1979) (Figs. 227 and 228).

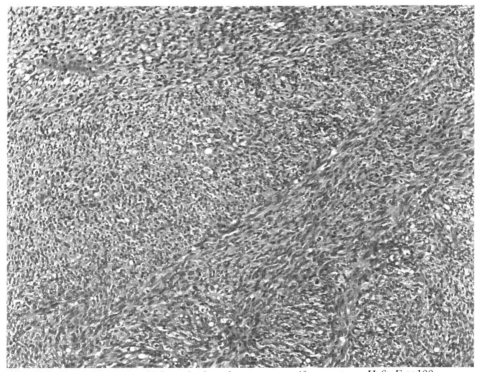

Fig. 224. Stromal sarcoma, high grade, homologous type, uniform pattern. H & E, ×100.

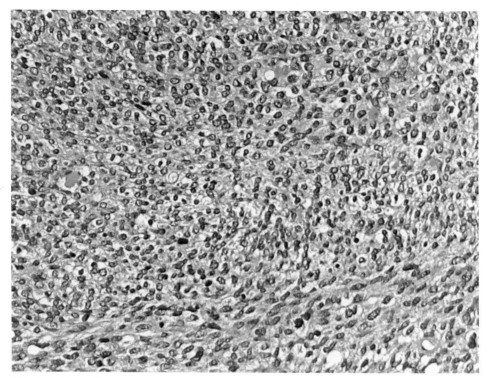

Fig. 225. Stromal sarcoma, high grade, homologous type, uniform pattern. H & E, ×250.

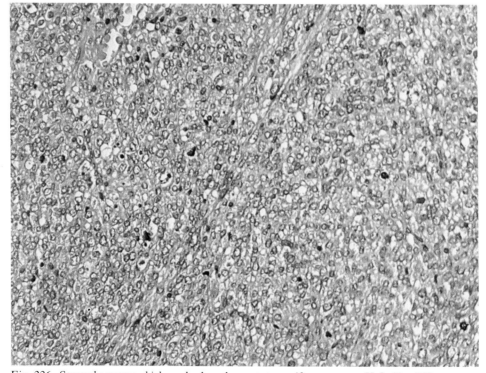

Fig. 226. Stromal sarcoma, high grade, homologous type, uniform pattern. H & E, ×250.

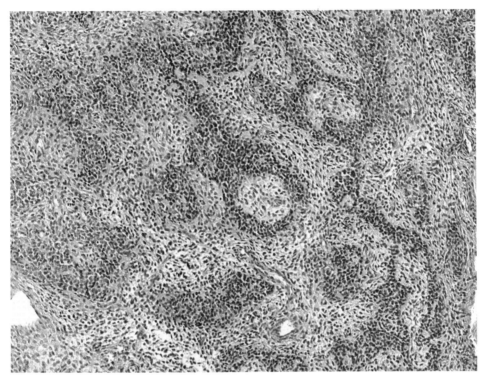

Fig. 227. Stromal sarcoma, high grade, homologous type, plexiform pattern. H & E, ×100.

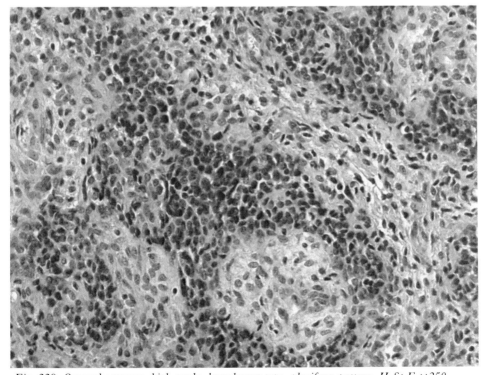

Fig. 228. Stromal sarcoma, high grade, homologous type, plexiform pattern. H & E, ×250.

The polymorphic type (Fig. 229 and 230): Shows a great variation in nuclear size, shape and chromatin density, mimicking the stromal differentiation into predecidual cells and endometrial granulocytes. There is a similar and corresponding variation in the amount of cytoplasm in these cells.

The malignant stromal cells of both types of stromal sarcoma grow destructively into the myometrium and infiltrate lymphatics and blood vessels (Fig. 229).

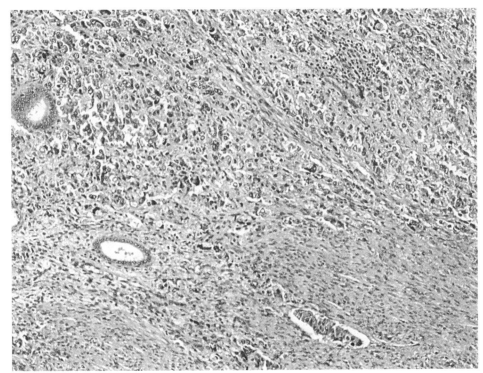

Fig. 229. Stromal sarcoma, high grade, polymorphic type. H & E, ×100.

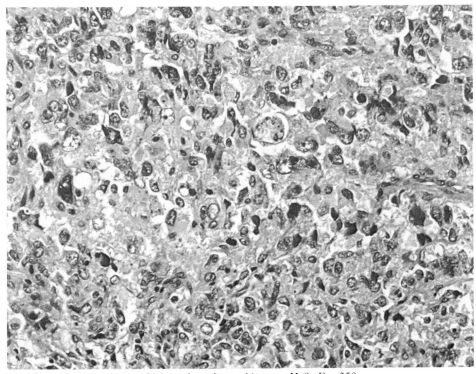

Fig. 230. Stromal sarcoma, high grade, polymorphic type. H & E, ×250.

Endolymphatic stromal myosis

(Figs. 231, 232 and 233). This is a low grade stromal sarcoma with the same cellular structure as the homologous type (Zaloudek and Norris 1982). The cells composing it differ from those of the homologous type only in their less pronounced mitotic activity, which is below 9 mitoses per 10 HPF. Characteristic of low grade stromal sarcoma is an early and extensive invasion of the lymphatic vascular spaces of the myometrium and penetration into tissue clefts of the myometrium without destruction and necrosis (Figs. 231 and 232). Whereas most of these low grade stromal sarcomas have a uniform pattern, a plexiform arrangement is occasionally seen (Clement and Scully 1976).

Morphologic differential diagnosis: a) Stromal nodule according to the criteria described above. b) Between high grade (uniform and polymorphic type) and low grade (endolymphatic stromal myosis) is possible according to two main criteria: mitotic activity (below or above 10 mitoses per 10 HPF) and mode of myometrial invasion (penetration or destruction).

Malignant mixed mesenchymal tumors

These rare tumors contain two or more types of sarcomatous tissues arriving from Müllerian epithelium with mesenchymal differentiation. Their morphology corresponds to the mesenchymal portions of malignant mixed Müllerian tumor (see p. 208).

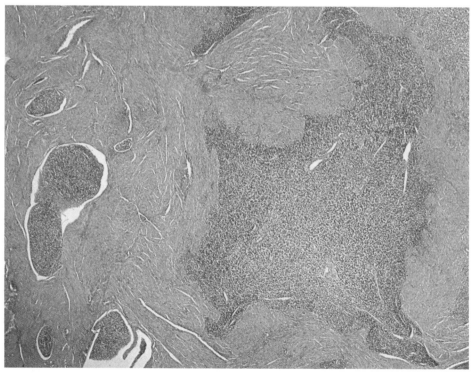

Fig.231. Endolymphatic stromal myosis (stromal sarcoma, low grade). H & E, ×25.

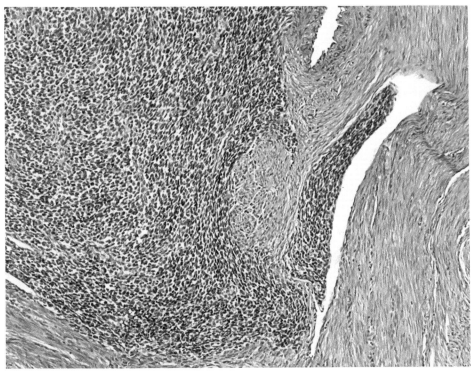

Fig. 232. Endolymphatic stromal myosis (stromal sarcoma, low grade). H & E,×100.

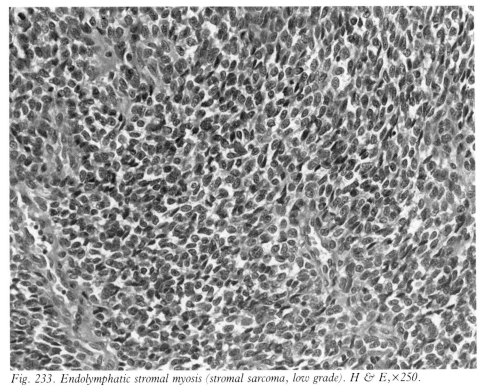

Fig. 233. Endolymphatic stromal myosis (stromal sarcoma, low grade). H & E,×250.

Mesodermal mixed tumors

These neoplasms contain both epithelial and mesenchymal elements which may be either uni- or pluripotential.

Papillary cystadenofibroma

(Figs. 234 and 235). This rare endometrial tumor (Vellios and Reagan 1973) is a benign variant of the malignant Müllerian mixed tumor. It consists of polypoid or lobular masses of long branching papillae which may fill out large portions of the uterine cavity. They are covered by a single row of low cuboidal or columnar epithelium and contain no or very few small resting or proliferating glands. Due to the profuse branching, buds of the epithelium become caught up in the stroma, forming gland-like structures. The stroma mainly consists of spindle-shaped fibroblasts occasionally separated by edema. Their nuclei are regular. Mitoses are rare. Cellular pleomorphism does not occur.

Morphologic differential diagnosis is possible from: a) Endometrial polyps: these lack the extensive branching, their stroma is less cellular and contains more endometrial glands. b) Homologous stromal sarcoma. This is not papillary and consists of poorly differentiated stromal cells with frequent mitoses. c) Adenosarcoma: this malignant variant of adenofibroma is characterized by focal (often periglandular) or diffuse stromal hypercellularity, where numerous stromal cells are found in mitosis.

The papillary cystadenofibroma may undergo various types and degrees of malignant change:

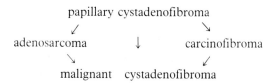

papillary cystadenofibroma

adenosarcoma   carcinofibroma

malignant cystadenofibroma

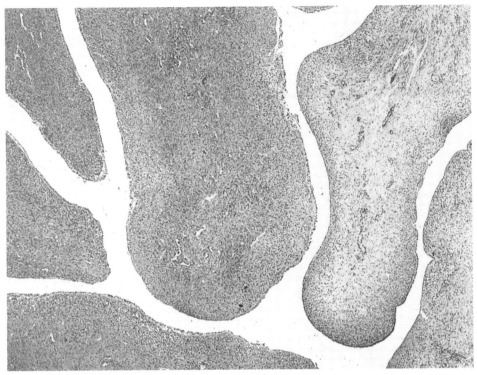

Fig. 234. Papillary cystadenofibroma. H & E, ×25.

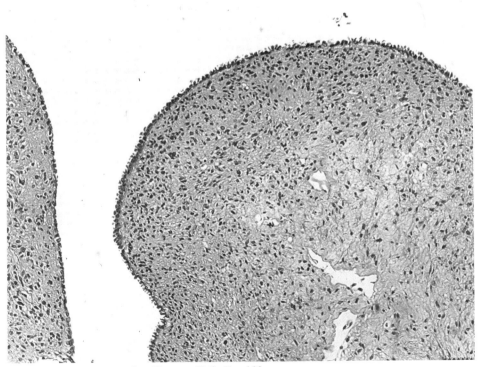

Fig. 235. Papillary cystadenofibroma. H & E, ×100.

199

Adenosarcoma

(Figs. 236, 237 and 238). The general structure and the epithelial component of this tumor closely resemble those of the benign adenofibroma. Some glandular spaces may be cystically dilated and contain mucin (Fig. 236). The mesodermal component, however, is more cellular and composed of small sarcomatous fibroblasts or stromal cells with mild atypia and moderate mitotic activity (Clement and Scully 1974; Zaloudek and Norris 1982). Characteristic are the round hypercellular foci forming perivascular nodules or periglandular cuffs (Czernobilsky et al. 1983) (Fig. 237).

Clinical correlation and morphologic differential diagnosis: a) Adenofibroma: patients with adenofibroma are generally older; their median age is approximately 68 years in comparison to 57 years for the patients with adenosarcoma (Zaloudek and Norris 1982). Mitotic activity is too variable to serve as a reliable diagnostic criterion. Focal stromal hypercellularity with pleomorphism is characteristic of adenosarcoma and absent in adenofibroma. Adenosarcomas do invade the myometrium, but only at a late stage. b) Stromal sarcoma: marked mitotic activity, absence of cleft-like spaces and cystic glands. Early destructive invasion of the myometrium with necrosis is characteristic of stromal sarcoma and absent in adenosarcoma.

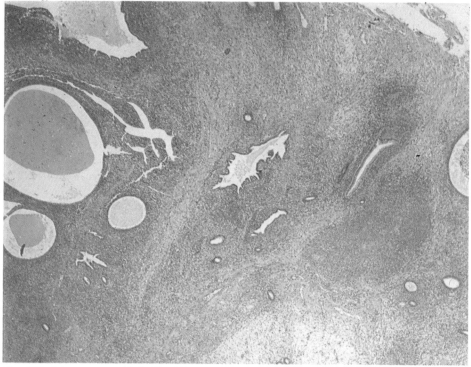

Fig. 236. Adenosarcoma. H & E, ×25.

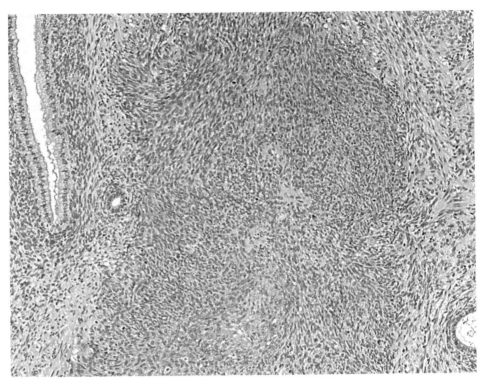

Fig. 237. Adenosarcoma. H & E, ×100.

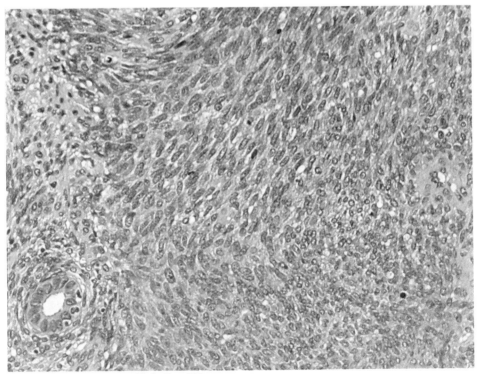

Fig. 238. Adenosarcoma. H & E, ×250.

Carcinofibroma

(Figs. 239 and 240). In these rare tumors, the epithelial component is malignant, whereas the mesenchymal component is benign (Östör and Fortune 1980). The epithelial component consists of carcinomatous glands which may be cystically dilated or microalveolar, and may form branching intraluminal epithelial papillae or nodules of squamous metaplasia (Fig. 239). The lining epithelium is atypical and resembles that of adenocarcinomas. The surrounding stroma corresponds to that of benign adenofibromas, consisting mainly of fibroblasts (Fig. 240). The tumor may invade the myometrium like an adenocarcinoma.

Morphologic differential diagnosis from adenocarcinoma with desmoplastic stromal reaction is possible because of the large amount of fibrous stroma resulting in a widely spaced arrangement of the carcinomatous glands.

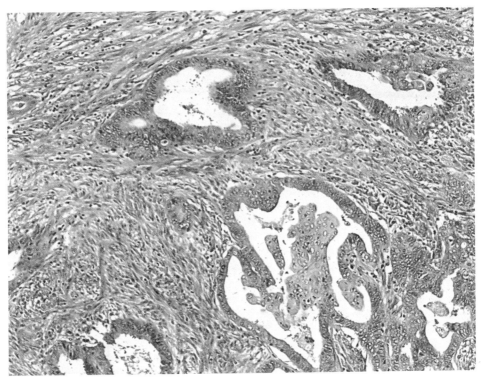

Fig. 239. Carcinofibroma. H & E, ×100.

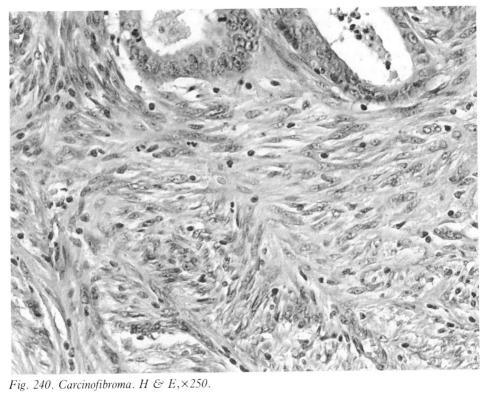

Fig. 240. Carcinofibroma. H & E, ×250.

Malignant papillary cystadenofibroma

(Figs. 241, 242 and 243). In this neoplasm both epithelial and mesenchymal components are malignant. In structure and arrangement the carcinomatous glands appear similar to those in carcinofibroma, and the sarcomatous stroma corresponds closely to that of an adenosarcoma. Occasional accumulations of clear cells surround cleft-like spaces or form larger sheets.

Morphologic differential diagnosis: This tumor is a special subtype of carcinosarcoma developing by malignant transformation of a benign adenofibroma, by carcinomatous change of an adenosarcoma or by sarcomatous change of a carcinofibroma. The characteristic original structure of the benign or low grade malignant precursor, in particular the branching papillae surrounding cleft-like spaces, can still be seen.

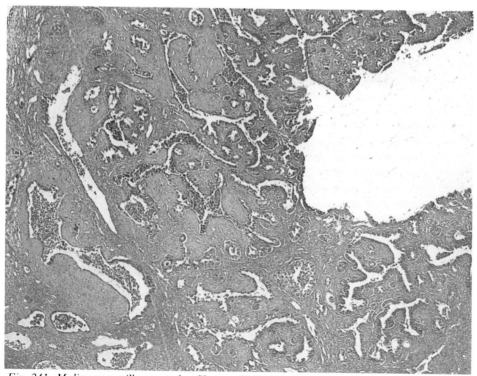

Fig. 241. Malignant papillary cystadenofibroma. H & E, ×25.

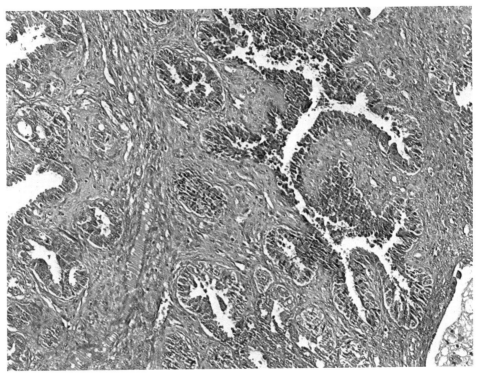

Fig. 242. Malignant papillary cystadenofibroma. H & E, ×100.

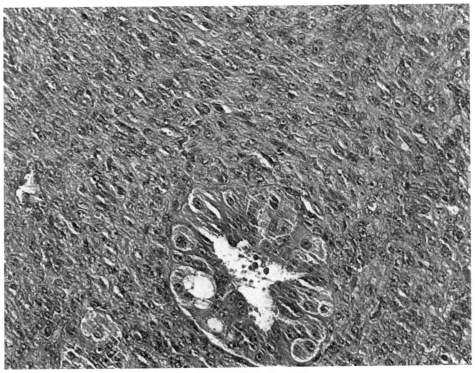

Fig. 243. Malignant papillary cystadenofibroma. H & E, ×250.

205

Carcinosarcoma

(Figs. 244, 245 and 246). This more frequent malignant mixed tumor grows more aggressively, fills the uterine cavity at an early stage and shows early myometrial and endocervical invasion. Histologically, the carcinomatous component closely resembles the endometrial or papillary type of adenocarcinoma with variously sized glands lined by atypical multilayered epithelial cells that form intraluminal branching papillae (Fig. 245). Occasional regions of clear cells or mucinous glands are common, whereas areas of squamous cell carcinoma are rare. The carcinomatous glands are widely separated by a sarcomatous stroma, which consists mostly of sarcomatous fibroblasts and endometrial stromal cells. Both components show frequent mitoses (Fig. 246). Hence, the sarcomatous component of carcinosarcoma, which is intimately admixed with the carcinomatous component, may be uniform or polymorphic, like an endometrial stromal sarcoma.

Morphologic differential diagnosis: a) Poorly differentiated adenocarcinoma, in which solid sheets of undifferentiated carcinomatous cells surround differentiated carcinomatous glands in a sarcomatoid pattern. The distinction is possible by careful study of the cellular structure, and by silver impregnation of the reticulin network: carcinomatous cells are enveloped by reticulin fibers in small groups, whereas sarcoma cells are enveloped individually, incompletely, or not at all. b) Malignant mixed Müllerian tumor: when the connective tissue component of the carcinosarcoma retains pluripotential qualities it may show heterotopic differentiation and produce cartilage, bone or striated muscle: it is then called a malignant mixed Müllerian tumor (see below).

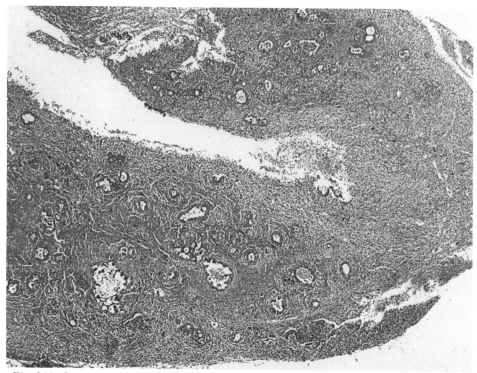

Fig. 244. Carcinosarcoma. H & E, ×25.

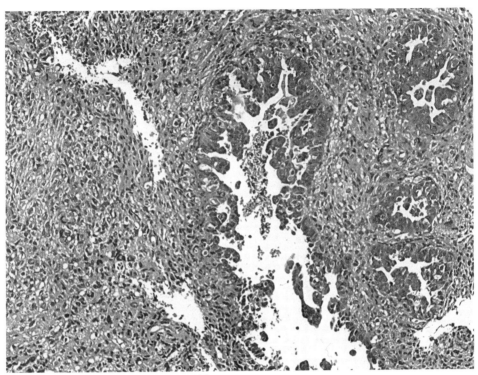

Fig. 245. Carcinosarcoma. H & E, ×100.

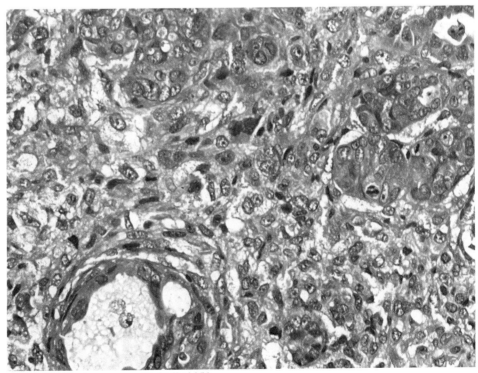

Fig. 246. Carcinosarcoma. H & E, ×250.

Malignant mixed Müllerian tumor

(Figs. 247-253). In this neoplasm the epithelial component corresponds closely to that seen in carcinosarcomas with fixed potentials, whereas the sarcomatous component may be extremely pleomorphic. Besides poorly differentiated mesenchymal cells and mingled with these one may find regions of atypical chondroblasts or osteoblasts (Figs. 247, 248 and 249). Cartilage is the second most common heterologous element in these tumors (Silverberg 1971). Other mixed tumors may contain large regions of rhabdomyoblasts with cross-striations (Böcker and Stegner 1975). When these elongated cells are cross-sectioned (cut at right angles to their long axis), their cross-striations cannot be seen and the cells appear round, surrounded by empty spaces (Figs. 250 and 251). Large cells with vacuolated cytoplasm (Fig. 251) may represent a liposarcomatous component, a relatively rare occurrence (Mortel et al. 1970). Very occasionally, ganglion cells may be found (Ruffolo et al. 1969). Some mesodermal mixed tumors contain large regions of a myxosarcoma (Fig. 252), others areas of a leiomyosarcoma (Fig. 253), which have to be differentiated from a pure myxosarcoma or leiomyosarcoma, respectively.

Morphologic differential diagnosis: Problems may arise only when insufficient tissue sections have been taken for study. To ensure that the wide spectrum of potentials of these mixed tumors is included, many sections should be studied from several different parts of the tumor. Under these circumstances, the differential diagnosis from other neoplasms proves to be an unrealistic problem.

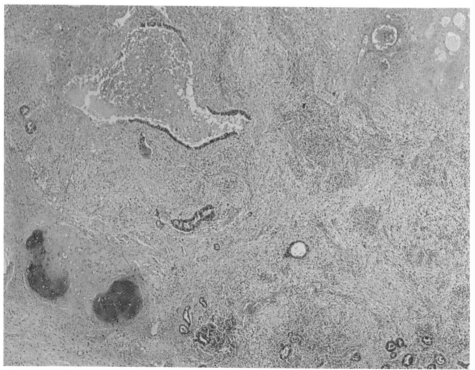

Fig. 247. Malignant mixed Müllerian tumor with chondroblasts. H & E, ×25.

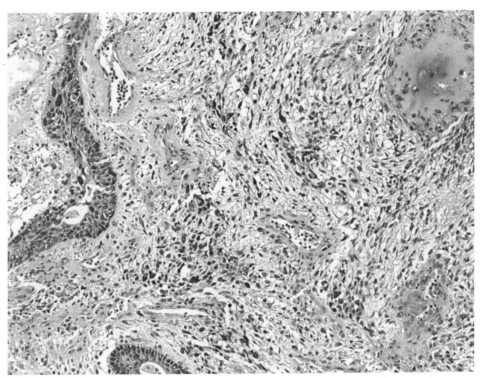

Fig. 248. Malignant mixed Müllerian tumor with chondroblasts. H & E, ×100.

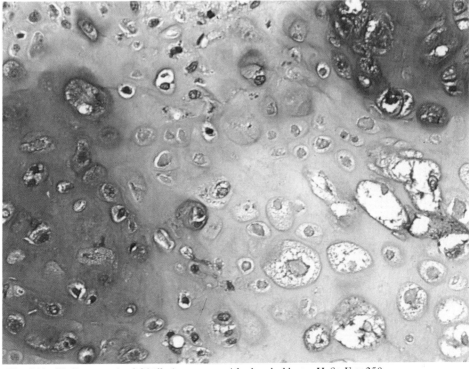

Fig. 249. Malignant mixed Müllerian tumor with chondroblasts. H & E, ×250.

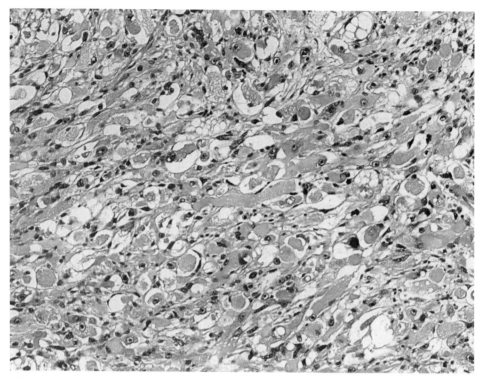

Fig. 250. Malignant mixed Müllerian tumor with rhabdomyoblasts. H & E,×100.

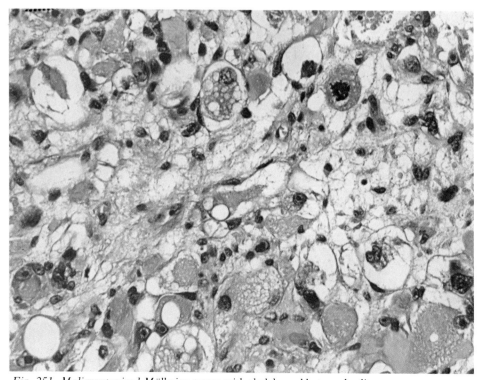

Fig. 251. Malignant mixed Müllerian tumor with rhabdomyoblasts and a liposarcomatous component. H & E,×250.

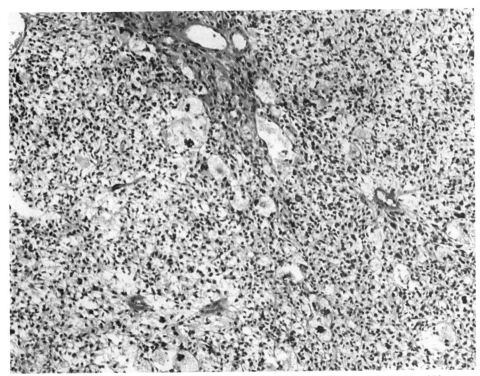

Fig. 252. Malignant mixed Müllerian tumor with regions of a myxosarcoma. H & E, ×100.

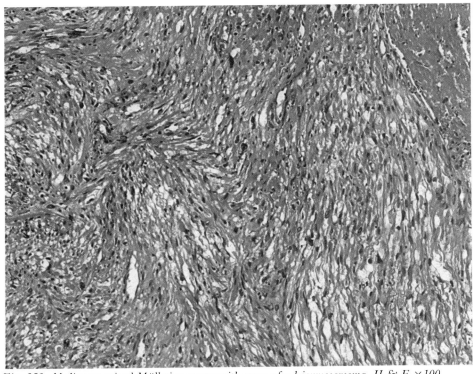

Fig. 253. Malignant mixed Müllerian tumor with areas of a leiomyosarcoma. H & E, ×100.

Secondary tumors

Carcinomas metastasizing to the endometrium most commonly originate in the cervix or ovaries, less commonly in the Fallopian tube, breast or gastrointestinal tract, and rarely in others organs. Whereas it may be difficult to distinguish a metastasis of a primary ovarian endometrioid carcinoma from a primary endometrial carcinoma, metastases from carcinomas structurally different from primary endometrial carcinomas can be easily recognized.

Metastases from primary breast carcinoma

(Figs. 254 and 255). The endometrial stroma is diffusely infiltrated and replaced in vast regions by large pleomorphic carcinomatous cells, many with a signet-ring form, typical of some primary carcinomas of the breast or gastrointestinal tract. Very few normal endometrial glands are preserved (Kjaer and Holm-Jensen 1972).

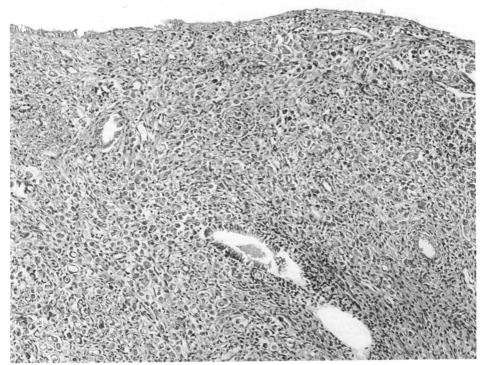

Fig. 254. Endometrial metastasis from primary breast carcinoma. H & E, ×100.

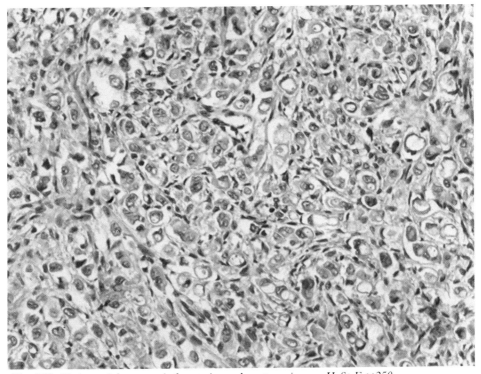

Fig. 255. Endometrial metastasis from primary breast carcinoma. H & E, ×250.

Endometrial involvement from primary carcinoma of the cervix

(Figs. 256 and 257). Invasion of the endometrium may occur through lymphatics or by continuous spread up the endocervical canal (Mitani et al. 1964). The surface epithelium is replaced by multilayered, dysplastic and atypical squamous epithelium which may invade the endometrium by plump or net-like infiltrations. The underlying stroma is densely cellular and contains chronic inflammatory infiltrates. Only very few narrow inactive endometrial glands may be preserved. If the atypical squamous epithelium shows a complete loss of stratification but is non-invasive it may have grown from a carcinoma in situ of the cervix (Kanbour and Stock 1978; Wilkinson et al. 1980).

Morphologic differential diagnosis is important from ichthyosis uteri which may also be dysplastic, but is in most instances a non-invasive metaplastic reaction of the superficial epithelium. If the ichthyosis overlies an invasive carcinoma, it should not be called ichthyosis any longer (cf. Fig. 55).

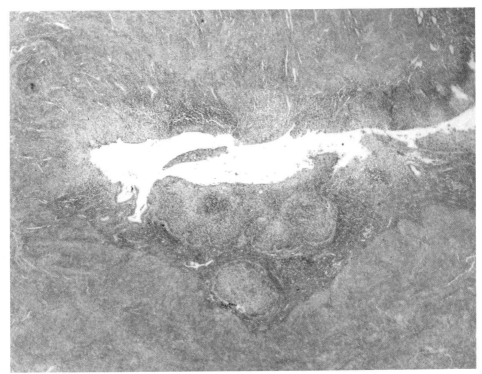

Fig. 256. Endometrial involvement from primary carcinoma of the cervix. H & E, ×25.

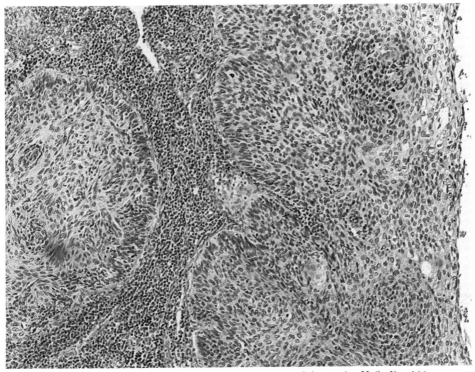

Fig. 257. Endometrial involvement from primary carcinoma of the cervix. H & E, ×100.

Leukemic infiltrations

(Figs. 258, 259 and 260). Characteristically the gross architecture of the endometrium remains preserved, making it difficult to recognize the leukemic infiltration under low magnification (Fig. 258).

At higher magnification (Figs. 259 and 260) a diffuse infiltration and often replacement of the endometrial stroma by leukemic cells becomes evident. Between these infiltrates, irregular hemorrhages can be seen (Fig. 259). The endometrial glands are in general preserved, most of them uninvolved, although a few may show infiltration by leukemic cells (Kapadia et al. 1978).

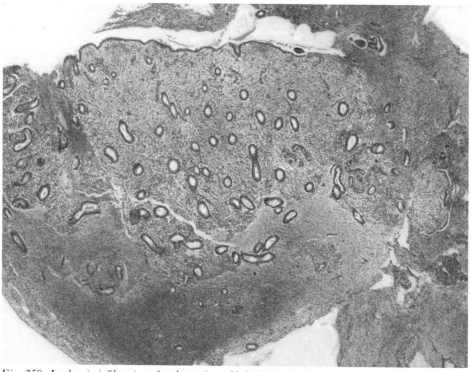

Fig. 258. Leukemic infiltration of endometrium. H & E, ×25.

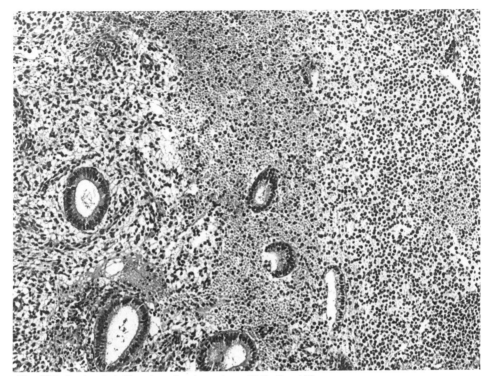

Fig. 259. Leukemic infiltration of endometrium. H & E, ×100.

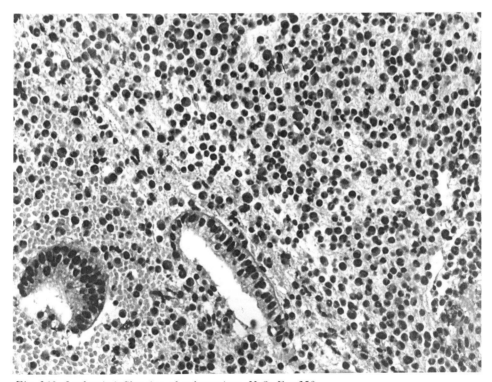

Fig. 260. Leukemic infiltration of endometrium. H & E, ×250.

Literature

Akhtar, M., Kim, P.Y. & Young, I.: Ultrastructure of endometrial stromal sarcoma. Cancer *35:* 406, 1975.

Ancla, M., de Brux, J., Musset, R. & Bret, J.A.: Etude au microscope électronique de l'endomètre humain dans différentes conditions d'équilibre hormonal. Arch. Path. *15:* 136, 1967.

Arias-Stella, J.: Atypical endometrial changes associated with the presence of chorionic tissue. Arch. Path. *58:* 112, 1954.

Böcker, W. & Stegner, H.-E.: Mixed Müllerian tumors of the uterus. Ultrastructural studies on the differentiation of rhabdomyoblasts. Virch. A. path. Anat. Histol. *863:* 337, 1975.

Charles, D.: Iatrogenic endometrial patterns. J.clin.Path. *17:* 205, 1964.

Christopherson, W.M., Alberhasky R.C. & Connelly, P.J.: Carcinoma of the endometrium: I. A clinicopathologic study of clear-cell carcinoma and secretory carcinoma. Cancer *49:* 1511, 1982 a.

Christopherson, W.M., Alberhasky, R.C. & Connelly, P.J.: Carcinoma of the endometrium. II. Papillary adenocarcinoma: A clinical pathological study of 46 cases. Am.J.clin.Path. *77:* 534, 1982 b.

Clement, P.B. & Scully, R.E.: Müllerian adenosarcoma of the uterus. Cancer *34:* 1138, 1974.

Clement, P.B. & Scully R.E.: Uterine tumors resembling ovarian sex-cord tumors. A clinicopathologic analysis of fourteen cases. Am. J. clin. Path. *66:* 512, 1976.

Connelly, P.J., Alberhasky, R.C. & Christopherson, W.M.: Carcinoma of the endometrium. III. Analysis of 865 cases of adenocarcinoma and adenoacanthoma. Obstet. Gynec. *59:* 569, 1982.

Czernobilsky, B., Hohlweg-Majert, P. & Dallenbach-Hellweg, G.: Uterine adenosarcoma: A clinicopathologic study of 11 cases with a reevaluation of histologic criteria. Arch. Gynec. *233:* 281, 1983.

Dallenbach, F.D. & Dallenbach-Hellweg, G.: Immunohistologische Untersuchungen zur Lokalisation des Relaxins in menschlicher Plazenta und Dezidua. Virshows Arch. path Anat. *337:* 301, 1964.

Dallenbach, F.D. & Dallenbach-Hellweg, G.: Fluoreszenzmikroskopische Tagesdiagnostik des menstruellen Zyklus und erste Anzeichen der senilen Involution. Verh. Dtsch. ges. Path. *52:* 342, 1968.

Dallenbach-Hellweg, G.: Über die Schaumzellen im Stroma des Endometriums: Vorkommen und histochemische Befunde. Virshows Arch. path. Anat. *338:* 51, 1964.

Dallenbach-Hellweg, G.: Histopathology of the Endometrium. Berlin: Springer, 1981.

Dallenbach-Hellweg, G.: Vorkommen und histologische Struktur des Adenokarzinoms der Zervixschleimhaut nach langjähriger Einnahme von Ovulationshemmern. Geburtsh. u. Frauenheilk. *42:* 249, 1982.

Dallenbach-Hellweg, G.: The endometrium of infertility. Path. Res. Pracht. *178:* 527, 1984.

Dallenbach-Hellweg, G. & Bornebusch, C.G.: Histologische Untersuchungen über die Reaktion des Endometrium bei der verzögerten Abstoßung. Arch. Gynäk. *208:* 235, 1970.

Dallenbach, F.D. & Rudolph, E.: Foam cells and estrogen activity of the human endometrium. Arch. Gynäk. *217:* 335, 1974.

Dallenbach-Hellweg, G., Weber, J., Stoll, P. & Velten, C.H.: Zur Differentialdiagnose adenomatöser Endometriumhyperplasien junger Frauen. Arch. Gynäk. *210:* 303, 1971.

Daly, J.J. & Balogh, K.: Hemorrhagic necrosis of the senile endometrium ("Apoplexia uteri"). New Engl. J. Med. *278:* 709, 1968.

Eichner, E. & Abellera, M.: Endometrial hyperplasia treated by progestins. Obstet. Gynec. *38:* 739, 1971.

Fechner, R.E. & Kaufman, R.H.: Endometrial adenocarcinoma in Stein-Leventhal Syndrome. Cancer *34:* 444, 1974.

Fechner R.E., Bossart, M.I. & Spjut, H.J.: Ultrastructure of endometrial stromal foam cells. Am. J. clin. Pathol. *72:* 628, 1979.

Ferenczy, A.: Studies of the cytodynamics of human endometrial regeneration. Amer. J. Obstet. Gynec. *124:* 64, 582, 1976.

Fettig, O.: ^{3}H-Index-Bestimmungen und Berechnungen der mittleren Generationszeit (Lebensdauer) der Einzelabschnitte des gesunden und krankhaften Endometriums nach autoradiographischen Untersuchungen mit ^{3}H-Thymidin. Arch. Gynäk. *200:* 659, 1965.

Filippe, M.I. & Dawson, I.M.P.: Qualitative and quantitative enzyme histochemistry of the human endometrium and cervix in normal and pathological conditions. J. Path. Bact. *95:* 243, 1968.

Flowers, C.E. & Wilborn, W.H.: New observations on the physiology of menstruation. Obstet. Gynec. *51:* 16, 1978.

Fuchs, M.: Über die "hellen Zellen" im Epithel der menschlichen Uterusschleimhaut. Acta. anat. (Basel) *39:* 244, 1959.

Gigon, U., Herzer, H., Stamm, O. & Zarro, D.: Endometriumveränderung und luteotrope Sekretionsanomalien bei Gelbkörperinsuffizienz. Z. Geburtsh. Gynäk. *173:* 304, 1970.

Goldberg, B & Jones, H.W.: Acid phosphatase of the endometrium. Histochemical demonstration in various normal and pathologic conditions. Obstet. Gynec. *7:* 542, 1956.

Gore, B.Z. & Gordon, M.: Fine structure of epithelial cell of secretory endometrium in unexplained primary infertility. Fertil. and Steril. *25:* 103, 1974.

Gross, S.J.: Ribonucleoprotein, glucuronidase, and phosphamidase in normal and abnormal endometrium. Amer. J. Obstet. Gynec. *90:* 166, 1964.

Gusberg, S.B. & Hall, R.E.: Precursors of corpus cancer. III. The appearance of cancer of the endometrium in estrogenically conditioned patients. Obstet. Gynec. *17:* 397, 1961.

Hamperl, H.: Über die endometrialen Granulozyten (endometriale Körnchenzellen). Klin. Wschr. *32:* 665, 1954.

Hanson, D.J.: Studies of the endometrial stroma in cystic glandular hyperplasia. Amer. J. clin. Path. *32:* 152, 1959.

Hellweg, G.: Über endometriale Körnchenzellen (endometriale Granulozyten). Arch. Gynäk. *185:* 150, 1954.

Hempel, E., Böhm, W., Carol, W. & Klinger, G.: Zur Problematik von Bestimmung und Beurteilung der Östrogen-Aufbaudosis am menschlichen Endometrium. Zbl. Gynäk. *99:* 1060, 1977.

Henzl, M., Jirasek, J. Horsky, J. & Presl, J.: Die Proliferationswirkung des 17-α-Äthinyl-19-Nor-Testosteron. Arch. Gynäk. *199:* 335, 1964.

Holmstrom, E.G. & McLennan, C.E.: Menorrhagia associated with irregular shedding of the endometrium. Amer. J. Obstet. Gynec. *53:* 727, 1947.

Horie, A., Yasumoto, K., Ueda, H., Watanabe, Y., Kotoo, Y. & Kurita, Y.: Clear cell adenocarcinoma of the uterus-ultrastructural and hormonal study. Acta path. jap. *27:* 907, 1977.

Hughes, E.C., Jacobs, R.D. & Rubulis, A.: Effect of treatment for sterility and abortion upon the carbohydrate pathways of the endometrium. Amer. J. Obstet. Gynec. *89:* 69, 1964.

Johannisson E., Landgren, B.-M. & Hagenfeldt, M.D.: The effect of intrauterine progesterone on the DNA-content in isolated human endometrial cells. Acta cytol. *21:* 441, 1977.

John, H.A., Cornes, J.S. Jackson, W.D. & Bye, P.: Effect of a systemically administered progesterone on histopathology of endometrial carcinoma. J. Obstet. Gynac. Brit. Cwlth. *81:* 786, 1974.

Kanbour, A. & Stock, J.: Squamous cell carcinoma in situ of the endometrium and fallopian tube as superficial extension of invasive cervical carcinoma. Cancer *42:* 570, 1978.

Kapadia, S.B., Krause, J.R., Kanbour, A.I. & Hartstock, R.J.: Granulocytic sarcoma of the uterus. Cancer *41:* 687, 1978.

Kistner, R.W.: Histological effects of progestins on hyperplasia and carcinoma in situ of the endometrium. Cancer (Philad.) *12:* 1106, 1959.

Kistner, R.W., Griffiths, C.T. & Craig, J.M.: Use of progestional agents in the management of endometrial cancer. Cancer (Philad.) *18:* 1563, 1965.

Kjaer, W. & Holm-Jensen, S.: Metastases to the uterus. Acta path. microbiol. scand. A *80:* 835, 1972.

Komorowski, R.A., Garancis, J.C. & Clowry, L.J.: Fine structure of endometrial stromal sarcoma. Cancer *26:* 1042, 1970.

Kurman, R.J. & Norris, H.J.: Evaluation of criteria for distinguishing atypical endometrial hyperplasia from well-differentiated carcinoma. Cancer *49:* 2547, 1982.

Kurman, J. & Scully, R.E.: Clear cell carcinoma of the endometrium. An analysis of 21 cases. Cancer (Philad.) *37,* 872, 1976.

Lewin, E.: Histochemische Untersuchungen an Uterusschleimhäuten. Z. Geburtsh. Gynäk. *157:* 196, 1961.

Lomax, C.W., Harbert, G.M. & Thornton, W.N.: Actinomycosis of the female genital tract. Obstet. Gynec. *48:* 341, 1976.

McKay, D.G., Hertig, A.T., Bardawil, W. & Velardo, J.T.: Histochemical observations on the endometrium: I. Normal endometrium. II. Abnormal endometrium. Obstet. Gynec. *8:* 22, 140, 1956.

Mitani, Y., Yukimari, S., Jimi, S. & Jwasaki, H.: Carcinomatous infiltration into the uterine body in carcinoma of the uterine cervix. Amer. J. Obstet. Gynec. *89:* 984, 1964.

Moricard, R.: Critères morphologiques utérines et vaginaux de l'exploration cytohormonale dans la phase lutéale. In: Colloques sur "La fonction lutéale". Paris: Masson & Cie. 1954.

Mortel, R., Nedwich, A., Lewis, G.C. & Brady, L.W.: Malignant mixed Müllerian tumors of the uterine corpus. Obstet. Gynec. *35:* 468, 1970.

Moukhtar, M., Aleem, F.A., Hung, H.C., Sommers, S.C., Klinger, H.P. & Romney, S.L.: The reversible behavior of locally invasive endometrial carcinoma in a chromosomally mosaic. Cancer *40:* 2957, 1977.

Nogales, F., Martinez, H. & Parache, J.: Abstossung und Wiederaufbau des menschlichen Endometriums. Gynäk. Rundsch. *7:* 292, 1969.

Nogales-Ortiz, F., Puerta, J. & Nogales, F.F.: The normal menstrual cycle. Chronology and mechanism of endometrial desquamation. Obstet. Gynec. *51:* 259, 1978.

Nordqvist, S.: Hormone effects on carcinoma of the human uterine body studied in organ culture. Acta obstet. gynec. scand *43:* 296, 1964.

Norris, H.J. & Taylor, H.B.: Mesenchymal tumors of the uterus. I. A clinical and pathological study of 53 endometrial stromal tumors. Cancer (Philad.) *19:* 755, 1966.

Noyes, R.W., Hertig, A.T. & Rock, J.: Dating the endometrial biopsy. Fertil. and Steril. *1:* 3, 1950.

Ober, W.B.: Synthetic progestagen-estrogen preparations and endometrial morphology. J. clin. Path. *19:* 138, 1966.

Ober, W.B.: Effects of oral and intrauterine administration of contraceptives on the uterus. Hum. Path. *8:* 513, 1977.

Östör, A.G. & Fortune, D.W.: Benign and low grade variants of mixed Müllerian tumor of the uterus. Histopathology *4:* 369, 1980.

Pepler, W.J. & Fouche, W.: Spontaneous polyovulation in the human and its effect on the endometrial pattern. S. Afr. J. Obstet. Gynaec. *6:* 50, 1968.

Philippe, E., Ritter, J., Renaud, R. & Gandar, R.: Le cycle endométrial normal biphasique. Rev. franç. Gynéc. *60:* 405, 1965.

Philippe, E. Ritter, J. & Gandar, R.: L'endomètre biphasique normal en période menstruelle. Gynéc. Obstét. *65:* 515, 1966.

Poulsen, H.E., Taylor, C.W. & Sobin, L.: Histological Typing of Female Genital Tract Tumours. Geneva: WHO. 1975.

Robboy, S.J. & Bradley, R.: Changing trends and prognostic features in endometrial cancer associated with exogenous estrogen therapy. Obstet. Gynec. *54:* 269, 1979.

Rock, J. & Hertig, A.T.: Information regarding the time of human ovulation derived from a study of 3 unfertilized and 11 fertilized ova. Amer. J. Obstet. Gynec. *47:* 343, 1944.

Rorat, E., Ferenczy, A. & Richart, R.M.: The ultrastructure of clear cell adenocarcinoma of endometrium. Cancer *33:* 880, 1974.

Rosado, A., Hernández, O., Aznar, R. & Hicks, J.J.: Comparative glycolytic metabolism in the normal and in the Copper treated human endometrium. Contraception *13:* 17, 1976.

Roth, L.M.: Clear cell adenocarcinoma of the female genital tract. Cancer *33:* 990, 1974.

Ruffolo, E.H., Metts, N.B. & Sanders, H.L.: Malignant mixed Müllerian tumors of the uterus: A clinicopathologic study of 9 patients. Obstet. Gynec. *33:* 544, 1969.

Schmidt-Matthiesen, H.: Die dysfunktionelle uterine Blutung. Histochemie und Mechanismus. Gynaecologia (Basel) *160:* 197, 1965.

Sengel, A. & Stoebner, P.: Ultrastructure de l'endomètre humain normal. Z. Zellforsch. *109:* 245, 260, 1970.

Silverberg, S.G.: Malignant mixed mesodermal tumor of the uterus: an ultrastrustural study. Amer. J. Obstet. Gynec. *110:* 702, 1971.

Silverberg, S.G. & De Giorgi, L.S.: Clear cell carcinoma of the endometrium. Cancer *31:* 1127, 1973.

Spechter, H.J.: Über die Deziduabildung ohne Schwangerschaft. Münch. med. Wschr. *982,* 1953.

Tang, C., Toker, C. & Ances, I.G.: Stromomyoma of the uterus. Cancer *43:* 308, 1979.

Tavassoli, F.A. & Norris, H.J.: Mesenchymal tumors of the uterus. VII. A clinicopathologic study of 60 endometrial stromal nodules. Histopathology *5:* 1, 1981.

Toth, F., Gimes, R., Horn, B. & Kerenyi, T.: Suche neuer Wege mit "low dose" Kontrazeptivmitteln. Z. ärztl. Fortbild. *66:* 957, 1972.

Vellios, F., Ng, A.B.P. & Reagan, J.W.: Papillary adenofibroma of the uterus A benign mesodermal mixed tumor of Müllerian origin. Amer. J. Clin. Path. *39:* 496, 1973.

Verhagen, A. & Themann, H.: Elektronenmikroskopische Untersuchungen am menschlichen Endometrium unter Einwirkung von Ovulationshemmern mit gleichzeitiger Oestrogen- und Gestagenwirkung. Arch. Gynäk. *209:* 162, 1970.

Wagner, D., Richart, R.M. & Terner, J.Y.: Deoxyribonucleic acid content of precursors of endometrial carcinoma. Cancer (Philad.) *20:* 1067, 1967.

Wan, L.S., Hsu, Y.-C., Ganguly, M. & Bigelow, B.: Effects of the Progestasert on the menstrual pattern, ovarian steroids and endometrium. Contraception *16:* 417, 1977.

Wilkinson, E.J., Andrasko, K.P. & Stafl, A.: Endometrial involvement by cervical intraepithelial neoplasia. Obstet. Gynec. *55:* 378, 1980.

Wilson, E.W.: The effect of copper on lactic dehydrogenase isoenzymes in human endometrium. Contraception *16:* 367, 1977.

Wynn, R.M.: Fine structural effects of intrauterine contraceptives on the human endometrium. Fertil. and Steril. *19:* 867, 1968.

Zaloudek, C.J. & Norris, H.J.: Mesenchymal tumors of the uterus. Progr. surg. Path. *3:* 1, 1982.

Index*

* Principal references are indicated by italicized numerals, and numbers in brackets refer to illustrations.